OXFORD MEDICAL PUBLICATIONS

Valvular Heart Disease

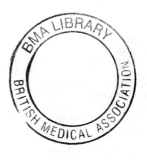

Oxford Specialist Handbooks in Cardiology

Valvular Heart Disease

Jim Newton

Nikant Sabharwal

Saul Myerson

Stephen Westaby

Bernard Prendergast

Department of Cardiology,
John Radcliffe Hospital,
Oxford, UK

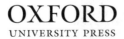

OXFORD
UNIVERSITY PRESS

OXFORD
UNIVERSITY PRESS

Great Clarendon Street, Oxford OX2 6DP.

Oxford University Press is a department of the University of Oxford.
It furthers the University's objective of excellence in research, scholarship,
and education by publishing worldwide in

Oxford New York

Auckland Cape Town Dar es Salaam Hong Kong Karachi
Kuala Lumpur Madrid Melbourne Mexico City Nairobi
New Delhi Shanghai Taipei Toronto

With offices in

Argentina Austria Brazil Chile Czech Republic France Greece
Guatemala Hungary Italy Japan Poland Portugal Singapore
South Korea Switzerland Thailand Turkey Ukraine Vietnam

Oxford is a registered trade mark of Oxford University Press
in the UK and in certain other countries

Published in the United States
by Oxford University Press Inc., New York

© Oxford University Press, 2011

The moral rights of the author have been asserted
Database right Oxford University Press (maker)

First published 2011

British Library Cataloguing in Publication Data
Data available

Library of Congress Cataloging-in-Publication-Data
Data available

Typeset by Glyph International, Bangalore, India
Printed in China
on acid-free paper through
Asia Pacific Offset

ISBN 978-0-19-955923-7

10 9 8 7 6 5 4 3 2 1

Foreword

This handbook on valvular heart disease is of interest to the reader because valve disease is an increasingly important health problem due to the increase in degenerative valve disease with the aging of the population. It is also a dynamic field due to the continuing improvements in diagnosis, especially imaging techniques, and treatment with the refinement of cardiac surgery but also the advent of percutaneous alternatives.

The chapters in this handbook separately cover each native valve disease, then the specific problem of patients with previous cardiac surgery which is increasingly frequent, and finally acute endocarditis.

For each chapter the handbook provides a comprehensive and critical "A-Z" review starting with pathophysiology and anatomy which are key for understanding imaging and treatment; then a large place is given to clinical examination, which is the first step of diagnosis and evaluation; the following step is a comprehensive description of echocardiography and other imaging techniques including the technical aspects, the most common pitfalls and finally the strategy of use; the treatment part includes medical treatment which plays an important role in endocarditis but essentially focuses on surgical techniques of valve replacement and repair and finally percutaneous techniques starting with the established ones such as percutaneous balloon mitral commissurotomy and giving a taste of the first results of percutaneous aortic valve implantation. At the end, recommendations for strategies are given largely based on the European Society of Cardiology guidelines.

The handbook is well-written, easy to read and its user-friendliness is aided by the large number of high quality illustrations especially on imaging. In conclusion, the group of authors led by Bernard Prendergast and colleagues should be congratulated for their efforts which will no doubt be highly appreciated by all the physicians and senior trainees who have an interest in cardiology.

Professor Alec Vahanian
Service de Cardiologie
Hôpital Bichat
Paris
France

August, 2010

Preface

Valvular heart disease is common and will become even more so as the population ages. The fall in the prevalence of rheumatic heart disease has changed the epidemiology of valvular heart disease and emerging technologies such as transcatheter valve implantation have revolutionized treatment in high risk patients. Echocardiography remains the main investigation for confirmation of diagnosis and assessment of severity, but it should be remembered that a full and careful history and clinical examination are essential in guiding management.

This handbook is aimed at trainee cardiologists, general physicians, cardiac surgeons, and related professional groups and covers the anatomy and pathophysiology of valvular heart disease before addressing each specific valve lesion in detail. Separate chapters on valve surgery, pregnancy, non-cardiac surgery, and infective endocarditis cover additional challenges in patients with valvular heart disease. Where applicable we have adhered to current European Society of Cardiology guidelines on the management of valvular heart disease and infective endocarditis, and have included an appendix of selected references.

JN
NS
SM
SW
BP

Contents

Symbols and abbreviations

📖	cross reference
AC	anterolateral commissure
ACE	angiotensin-converting enzyme
AR	aortic regurgitation
AS	aortic stenosis
AV	aortic valve
AVR	aortic valve replacement
BNP	brain natriuretic peptide
BSA	body surface area
CABG	coronary artery bypass grafting
CMR	cardiac magnetic resonance
CT	computed tomography
CXR	chest X-ray
ECG	electrocardiogram
EF	ejection fraction
EROA	effective regurgitant orifice area
FFP	fresh frozen plasma
HIV	human immunodeficiency virus
IE	infective endocarditis
INR	international normalised ratio
IV	intravenous
LV	left ventricle/ventricular
LVEDD	left ventricular end diastolic diameter
LVEDS	left ventricular end systolic diameter
LVOT	left ventricular outflow tract
MR	mitral regurgitation
MS	mitral stenosis
P½t	pressure half time
PC	postero-lateral commissure
PCC	prothrombin complex concentrate
PICC	peripherally inserted central venous catheter
PISA	proximal isovelocity surface area
PR	pulmonary regurgitation
PS	pulmonary stenosis
RA	right atrium

RV	right ventricle/ventricular
SAM	systolic anterior motion
TAPSE	tricuspid annular plane systolic excursion
TAVI	transcatheter aortic valve implantation
TOE	transoesophogeal echocardiography
tPA	tissue plasminogen activator
TR	tricuspid regurgitation
TS	tricuspid stenosis
TTE	transthoracic echocardiography
VSD	ventricular septal defect
VTI	velocity time integral

Chapter 1

Introduction to valvular heart disease

Introduction

Valvular heart disease is common and increasing in prevalence with the increase in life expectancy. It requires careful assessment and management for appropriate treatment of the range of disease severity, from minor disease that requires little follow up to the more severe manifestations that frequently lead to surgical intervention. The patient populations of all forms of valvular heart disease are changing, with degenerative lesions now dominant as the incidence of rheumatic valve disease continues to fall.

The aging population also presents additional management challenges since these patients often have multiple co-morbidities and require complex multidisciplinary assessment and intervention. While there have been few changes in effective medical therapy, new surgical interventions and more recent transcatheter interventions are now available, further changing the treatment paradigm.

Despite the high prevalence of valvular heart disease and wide variety of therapeutic options, few randomised clinical trials exist: the majority of management recommendations are derived from international guidelines. There is, however, evidence that many patients with proven valvular heart disease do not receive optimal therapy, and this book aims to guide healthcare professionals in the delivery of optimal care.

Epidemiology

The prevalence of valvular heart disease is changing. Rheumatic lesions such as mitral stenosis (MS) are declining in developed countries whereas degenerative lesions such as aortic stenosis (AS) are becoming more common, due in part to the ageing population.

The overall prevalence of valvular heart disease in the general population is around 2%, with no difference between men and women but a marked increase in prevalence with age (0.7% in 18–44 year olds and 13.3% in those over 75 years old).

Worldwide differences

Europe

The frequencies of individual lesions in European patients with valvular heart disease are:

- Aortic stenosis   43%
- Mitral regurgitation   31%
- Aortic regurgitation   13%
- Mitral stenosis   12%
- Right sided lesions   1%

~20% of these patients have multiple valve lesions, usually left sided valvular heart disease with secondary right heart changes.

Developing countries

- Rheumatic valvular heart disease remains a major public health problem in developing countries. The incidence of rheumatic fever is 100 in 100,000 in the Sudan, compared to <1 in 100,000 in the West. The prevalence of chronic rheumatic heart disease is estimated to be between 2.7–14.3 per 1000 people.

Newer aetiologies

In recent decades, new forms of valvular heart disease have emerged:

Drug-related valvular heart disease

- Ergot alkaloid derivatives (e.g. methysergide and ergotamine) have been used to treat migraine, but can induce endocardial fibrosis and lead to valvular heart disease similar to that seen in the carcinoid syndrome.
- Fenfluramine and phentermine combination therapy was used to treat obesity in the early 1990s until numerous reports of excess regurgitant valve lesions emerged. The severity appears to relate to the duration and cumulative dose exposure of the drugs, which were subsequently withdrawn.

HIV-related valvular heart disease

- Rare—myocardial and pericardial disease are more common, unless a predisposing factor is present e.g. intravenous (IV) drug use.
- Infective endocarditis (IE) may involve atypical organisms or fungal disease.
- Sterile vegetations on cardiac valves are seen in some patients, similar to classical marantic endocarditis in malignancy. The incidence is around 5%. These lesions occasionally cause embolic events and can lead to diagnostic uncertainty at the time of echocardiography.

Novel idiopathic valvular heart disease

- Systemic inflammatory diseases e.g. anti-phospholipid syndrome can cause valvular heart disease, with regurgitant lesions seen in up to 35%.

Anatomy and pathophysiology

Valve anatomy

The diagnosis, assessment and management of any valve lesion are dependent on a clear understanding of the relevant anatomy of both the normal and diseased valve. All four cardiac valves are intimately related to the central fibrous skeleton of the heart (see Fig. 1.1). Note also the close relationship of the coronary arteries, coronary sinus and conduction system.

Natural history

The majority of valve lesions are chronic and slowly progressive with a long asymptomatic phase. The cardiac remodelling that occurs in response is compensatory and aims to maintain normal cardiac output at rest and on exertion. Eventually, these compensatory mechanisms fail and symptoms arise, initially with exercise and later at rest.

The major challenge in the management of valvular heart disease is the timing of intervention. Detection of the lesion in the asymptomatic phase is preferable to allow close monitoring and patient education to ensure subsequent early detection of decompensation and/or symptoms. Initial symptoms may be subtle as many patients are elderly and attribute their fatigue or dyspnoea to ageing or co-morbidity. Careful questioning and objective assessment of exercise capacity may be required.

The importance of early symptom detection

Survival in asymptomatic valvular heart disease is excellent but declines rapidly as decompensation and symptoms occur. For example, the risk of sudden death in asymptomatic severe AS is less than 1% but the average survival of severe AS with heart failure is less than one year.

Effect on the cardiovascular system

The effect of any individual valve lesion on the cardiovascular system is dependent on a number of factors:
- Dominant lesion—regurgitant or stenotic
- Speed of onset—acute vs. chronic
- Underlying cardiac disease—e.g. ischaemia
- Pre-existing left ventricular (LV) hypertrophy—hypertension
- Arrhythmia—e.g. atrial fibrillation
- Co-morbidity—e.g. pulmonary disease affecting right heart lesions.

The adaptive responses of the ventricle are well described. Understanding the effects of the valve lesion and secondary cardiac changes aids understanding of the benefits and limitations of medical and surgical therapy.

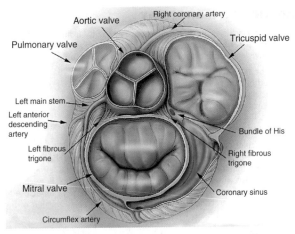

Fig. 1.1 Relationship of the four cardiac valves and other important cardiac structure. Reproduced with permission from Verma S., Mesana T.G. (2009) Mitral-Valve Prolapse *NEJM 361: 2261–2269*. ©2009 Massachusetts Medical Society. All rights reserved.

Regurgitant lesions

The cardiac response to regurgitant lesions is very different for acute and chronic disease. Chronic lesions progress slowly, with volume loading of the ventricle leading to progressive dilation and increased stroke volume to compensate for the regurgitation.

Acute regurgitation typically leads to abrupt decompensation since the ventricle has not had sufficient time to adapt to the changing haemodynamics. There are limited ways to respond and this is usually through increased heart rate. Urgent surgical intervention is often required.

Stenotic lesions

Obstruction to ventricular outflow leads to adaptive hypertrophy of the ventricle to maintain adequate driving pressure. This ultimately leads to decompensation and ventricular failure. Stenotic atrioventricular valves primarily lead to changes in the atrium but ultimately affect ventricular filling with resultant heart failure.

Aortic valve anatomy

The aortic valve is a trileaflet valve separating the LV from the aorta. It is an integral part of the aortic root and also closely related to the anterior mitral valve leaflet and the membranous ventricular septum.

The aortic valve complex consists of:
- LV outflow tract
- Aortic annulus
- Semilunar valve leaflets
- Interleaflet triangles
- Sinuses of Valsalva and sinotubular junction.

Left ventricular outflow tract

The outflow of the LV is bordered by the smooth curve of the ventricular septum and the aortic–mitral fibrous continuity joining the left and non-coronary cusps with the anterior (aortic) mitral valve leaflet. Between the right and non-coronary cusps lies the membranous septum; very close to the atrioventricular conduction bundle and the proximal portion of the left bundle (Fig. 1.2.).

Aortic annulus

The aortic annulus is a virtual ring at the base of the aortic valve (Fig. 1.3)— anatomically there is no distinct fibrous annulus at the junction between the ventricle and aorta. The posterior aspect of the aortic root (around the non-coronary leaflet) is largely fibrous whereas the remainder is ventricular muscle. A small amount of myocardium lies above what is considered the plane of the annulus, due to the semilunar attachments of the valve leaflets.

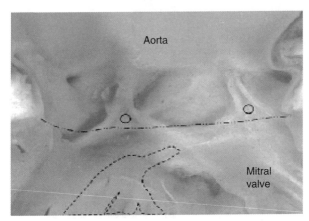

Fig. 1.2 The aortic root opened to demonstrate the three leaflets. The horizontal line demonstrates the ventriculo-arterial junction and the irregular shaped outline is the location of the conduction system and left bundle. Reproduced with permission from Ho S.Y. Structure and anatomy of the aortic root (2009) EJE 10:i3–i10, Oxford University Press.

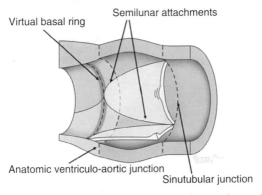

Fig. 1.3 Diagram of the aortic root demonstrating the semilunar attachments of each valve cusp and the difference in the true anatomical ventriculo-aortic junction and the 'virtual' aortic annulus. Reproduced with permission of the authors and the European Association for Cardio-Thoracic Surgery from: Anderson R.H. The surgical anatomy of the aortic root. Multimedia Man Cardiothorac Surg doi:10.1510/mmcts.2006.002527.

Aortic valve leaflets

The three semilunar leaflets (or cusps) of the aortic valve are conventionally described in relation to the coronary arteries:

- Left coronary cusp—situated below the left posterolateral sinus, from which the left main stem arises.
- Right coronary cusp—situated below the anterior sinus, from which the right coronary artery arises.
- Non-coronary cusp—situated below the right posterolateral sinus, also termed the 'non-facing' sinus as it is not adjacent to the pulmonary valve. There is no coronary artery arising from this sinus.

Each leaflet has a parachute-like shape and is attached to the aortic root along a semicircular line (Fig. 1.4). The three leaflet attachments meet at the level of the sinotubular junction and form the commissures. The leaflets are of roughly equal size, though there are small differences—the non-coronary leaflet is usually the largest of the three.

The surface area of the leaflets is around 40% greater than the area of the aortic root, allowing a significant area of leaflet apposition to withstand high aortic pressure. A thickened area at the midpoint of each leaflet corresponds to the point of leaflet apposition when closed. The height of the leaflets when open is lower than that of the sinuses to prevent obstruction of the coronary ostia.

Interleaflet triangles

The thin triangular areas between the valve leaflets, termed the trigones, project up into the aortic root from the true junction between the ventricular mass and aorta (Fig. 1.4). The interleaflet triangle between the right and non-coronary cusps joins the membranous septum to form the central fibrous body which is the landmark for the bundle of His.

As the collagen content of the interleaflet triangles is lower than the walls of the sinuses these are potential sites for dilation and aneurysm formation.

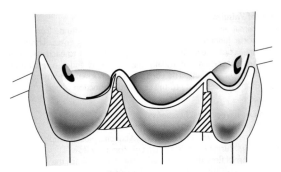

Fig. 1.4 The aortic root opened to demonstrate the three cusps, two coronary ostia and the interleaflet triangles (shaded). Reproduced from Underwood, M.J. et al. (2000) The aortic root: structure, function, and surgical reconstruction Heart; 83: 376–80 with permission from BMJ Publishing Group Ltd.

Sinuses of Valsalva

The proximal end of the aorta (the aortic root) extends from the ventricular-aortic junction to the more elastic ascending aorta. Three bulges of the aortic root, the sinuses of Valsalva, lie adjacent to each valve leaflet. The non-coronary sinus is usually slightly larger, and the left coronary sinus usually the smallest. The coronary ostia normally lie in the superior aspect of the sinuses, close to the sinotubular junction.

Function

The sinuses have several functions:
- Accommodation of the aortic leaflets when open, to allow unobstructed forward flow and avoid coronary obstruction
- Reservoirs during diastole to facilitate coronary flow
- Regulation of flow dynamics—eddy currents separate the leaflets from the aortic wall and aid prompt leaflet closure at the end of systole.

Sinotubular junction

The distal portion of the aortic root, where the sinuses meet the aorta, is the sinotubular junction. The aortic diameter at this point is typically ~75% of the maximal sinus diameter.

The sinotubular junction expands and contracts during the cardiac cycle, the diameter increasing in systole and reducing in diastole. The base of the root (the aortic annulus) decreases in size during systole, making the root more cylindrical and assisting forward flow. During diastole, the base and sinuses expand and the sinotubular junction contracts, forming a more conical aortic root and aiding leaflet closure.

Normal aortic valve physiology

The normal trileaflet aortic valve is relatively small, with an open area of 3–4cm^2 allowing free flow of blood out of the ventricle during systole. The high LV pressure facilitates flow across the aortic valve. In contrast flow across the mitral valve relies on a larger open leaflet area due to the low left atrial pressure. The aortic valve leaflets close just before the end of systole due to the dynamics of the sinuses and sinotubular junction, preventing regurgitation of blood from the aorta into the ventricle.

Normal values for the aortic root:
- Aortic annulus diameter*   1.4–2.6cm
- Aortic valve area   >2.0cm^2
- Ascending aorta diameter*   2.1–3.4cm
- Peak aortic velocity   <1.7m/s
- LV outflow tract velocity   0.7–1.1m/s

* Measurements of the annulus, sinus of Valsalva and sinotubular junction are best indexed to body surface area.

Aortic valve variations

While the normal aortic valve has three leaflets (Fig. 1.5), valves with one to five leaflets have been described. A bicuspid valve is by far the most common variant, being found in approximately 2% of the normal population.

Bicuspid valve

A bicuspid valve has variable anatomy depending on the leaflet configuration. The two most common types are:

• Two leaflets of roughly equal size (Fig. 1.6)
• One slightly larger leaflet (often with a central raphe) resulting from fusion of two smaller leaflets during development.

The typical configuration is for the two leaflets to be in an anterior–posterior configuration (effectively failure of separation of the right and left coronary cusps) with only 20% demonstrating a lateral orientation.

Associated aortic root dilation is not uncommon and related to coexisting abnormalities of the elastic lamina—these patients have a five-fold increase in the risk of aortic dissection (even after valve replacement).

Unicuspid valve

Rarely, a valve with a central orifice surrounded by a single circumferential leaflet is seen, usually in combination with left sided congenital malformations. This usually results in significant AS.

Quadricuspid/quinticuspid valve

These variants are rare and prone to regurgitation.

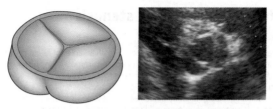

Fig. 1.5 Normal tricuspid aortic valve anatomy and appearance on transthoracic echocardiography.

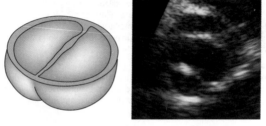

Fig. 1.6 Bicuspid aortic valve anatomy and appearance on transthoracic echocardiography.

Physiology of aortic stenosis

Effect on the left ventricle

The normal aortic valve has a maximal orifice area of $3-4cm^2$ which reduces as the valve becomes thickened and immobile, resulting in LV outflow obstruction and compensatory myocardial remodelling to maintain normal stroke volume. The LV hypertrophies becoming less compliant and diastolic filling is attenuated—atrial systole becomes increasingly important to maintain adequate filling and loss of atrial transport (associated with the onset of atrial fibrillation) can lead to a reduction in cardiac output and haemodynamic decompensation.

Progressive diastolic dysfunction is followed by increased wall stress and elevated afterload leading to chamber dilation and systolic dysfunction. Left untreated, progressive dilation and failure of the LV is inevitable. LV end-diastolic pressure climbs and pulmonary hypertension develops.

Some or all of these abnormalities may be reversible following relief of valve obstruction.

Myocardial ischaemia

Coronary perfusion can be impaired leading to ischaemia even when the coronary arteries are normal. This is due to the combination of increased LV pressure, reduced coronary perfusion pressure, and increased myocardial oxygen demand.

Syncope

Syncope is usually mediated by reduced cerebral perfusion as a consequence of arterial vasodilation without compensatory increase in cardiac output. It typically occurs during exertion and can also be mediated by an abnormal baroreceptor response to the increased systolic pressure of the LV.

General aspects of therapy

- The combination of a relatively fixed cardiac output with a ventricle dependent on adequate filling severely limits the role of medical therapy in AS. Vasodilators can cause hypotension and decompensation if not cautiously introduced, and while diuretics may relieve pulmonary congestion, excessive use can impair LV filling.
- β-blockers may be helpful to slow LV ejection and reduce myocardial work. They may also be useful for angina.
- Atrial fibrillation leading to decompensation should ideally be treated by restoring sinus rhythm if possible. Otherwise, rate control with digoxin or β-blockade is recommended.
- Some patients with AS and heart failure may benefit from very careful introduction of an ACE inhibitor under hospital supervision, if significant hypotension can be avoided.

Physiology of aortic regurgitation

Response of the ventricle

The early adaptive response of the ventricle is hypertrophy to preserve diastolic compliance and normalise wall stress and LV filling pressures. LV ejection fraction is maintained.

Persistent volume loading leads to progressive dilation of the LV to increase the stroke volume and compensate for the fall in net forward flow. Wall stress increases due to systemic hypertension. At this stage, LV function appears to be grossly normal.

If left untreated, LV dilation progresses further and systolic function starts to fail as the ventricle begins to decompensate. In addition, diastolic compliance falls due to diffuse myocardial fibrosis. This leads to an elevated LV end-diastolic pressure and eventual pulmonary oedema (Fig. 1.7).

Effect on blood pressure

In chronic aortic regurgitation (AR), adaptive dilation of the LV causes an increase in stroke volume to maintain net cardiac output. This increased stroke volume leads to systolic hypertension, while diastolic blood pressure is reduced as a result of the incompetent aortic valve. This leads to a wide pulse pressure, though the mean arterial pressure is often unchanged. This systolic hypertension should not be confused with hypertension from other causes and rarely needs treatment

General aspects of therapy

Medical therapy in AR is directed at reducing LV afterload and preload. Arterial vasodilators are used to lower afterload and reduce regurgitant flow by lowering the gradient across the regurgitant valve in diastole. Venodilators and diuretics lower LV preload and reduce both end-diastolic volume and pressure.

▶ Avoid rate-slowing drugs such as β-blockers, as these lengthen diastole and increase the total regurgitant volume. These agents are best avoided, even if systolic dysfunction has developed.

Acute aortic regurgitation

- In acute severe AR, the adaptive responses of the ventricle have not had time to occur and LV end diastolic pressure rises rapidly, with resultant pulmonary oedema.
- Systolic function is usually maintained but can decline rapidly.
- Vasodilator therapy to reduce afterload has a limited role in slowing deterioration but urgent definitive intervention (surgery) is required.

▶ The intra-aortic balloon pump should not be used as it increases diastolic pressure and exacerbates AR.

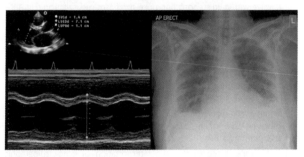

Fig. 1.7 The effects of aortic regurgitation. The left hand panel demonstrates a severely dilated left ventricle (M-mode echocardiography) and the right hand panel shows a chest X-ray of pulmonary oedema.

Mixed aortic valve disease

In patients with AS and AR, it is typical for one lesion to dominate and this usually drives the pathophysiological response—for example in dominant AS the LV exhibits hypertrophy rather than dilation.

If AR is moderate or worse, the additive effect on the stressed ventricle can precipitate pulmonary oedema even with non-severe AS. While the AS and AR may both be moderate and not require intervention in isolation, the combination may indicate earlier surgical treatment.

Combined valvular heart disease can also complicate assessment. A common misinterpretation is a high peak pressure drop across an aortic valve with mild stenosis but more significant regurgitation (Fig. 1.8). The increased stroke volume caused by the regurgitation leads to higher velocities across the valve. Using the continuity equation corrects this as the LV outflow stroke volume is also elevated (see 📖 p.62).

The clinical signs are driven by the dominant lesion:

Dominant aortic stenosis
• Small volume pulse
• Narrow pulse pressure.

Dominant aortic regurgitation
• Collapsing large volume pulse
• Wide pulse pressure.

Particular care is required in the interpretation of echocardiographic data. A hypertrophied ventricle without major dilation excludes chronic severe AR.

In difficult cases, earlier invasive assessment may be useful, although care is required when calculating valve area as the usual Fick method may underestimate valve area in the presence of significant AR.

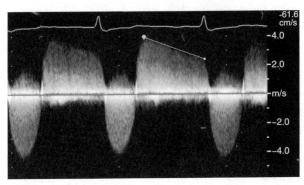

Fig. 1.8 Continuous wave Doppler in a case of mixed aortic valve disease with severe aortic stenosis and mild aortic regurgitation.

Mitral valve anatomy

The bileaflet left atrioventricular valve is named after its resemblance to a bishop's hat, or mitre, when open. Its twin functions are difficult to achieve, allowing unobstructed flow from the low pressure left atrium in ventricular diastole (requiring a large opening area), and resistance to high LV pressure during systole preventing regurgitation into the (low pressure) left atrium. To achieve this, the mitral valve consists of several interacting elements (Fig. 1.9) which form a complex unit, each with its own function.

- Mitral annulus
- Valve leaflets
- Chordae
- Papillary muscles
- LV wall.

Mitral annulus

As with all cardiac valves, there is no distinct ring shaped structure that the term 'annulus' suggests. The atrioventricular junction is variable in its composition and position. The anterior (aortic) portion is bordered by a straighter fibrous section including both the left and right fibrous bodies. The posterior portion is rounded and lacks fibrous tissue, rendering it more prone to dilation and calcification. The atrioventricular junction (annulus) does not lie on a flat plane, but is saddle shaped with compound curves (Fig. 1.10).

Changes in shape

The annulus is also a dynamic structure and varies in shape throughout the cardiac cycle. The overall area reduces by up to 40% during systole due to contraction of the ventricular muscle increasing the length of leaflet coaptation, which helps resist the high LV pressures.

The left atrial wall

The left atrial wall is in direct continuity with the posterior, or mural, leaflet of the mitral valve and the atrial myocardium forms part of the mitral annulus. Dilation of the atrium has potential to displace the mitral annulus with resultant mitral regurgitation (MR).

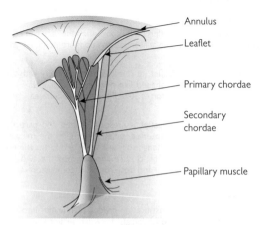

Fig. 1.9 The mitral valve complex demonstrating the annulus, leaflet, chordae and papillary muscle, and LV mass. Reproduced with permission from Verma S., Mesana T.G. (2009) Mitral-Valve Repair for Mitral-Valve Prolapse NEJM; 361:2261–2269. Copyright 2009 Massachusetts Medical Society. All rights reserved.

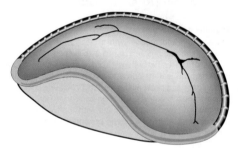

Fig. 1.10 Cartoon of the mitral annulus demonstrating its saddle shape with two 'peaks' and two 'valleys'.

Mitral leaflets

The two leaflets are very different. By convention they are named anterior and posterior, but their true anatomical positions are obliquely arranged.

Anterior leaflet

The 'anterior' or aortic leaflet (as it is in direct continuity with the aortic valve) is short and wide, shaped like a tongue. It occupies ~1/3 of the annular circumference but forms 50% of the total leaflet area.

Posterior leaflet

The 'posterior' or mural leaflet is crescent shaped and partially wraps round the 'tongue' of the anterior leaflet. It occupies the remaining two thirds of the annulus, being longer but less wide, and forms the remaining 50% of total leaflet area. The closure line between the two leaflets is curved, with an anterolateral and posteromedial commissure at each end (Fig. 1.11).

Leaflet scallops

The classical Carpentier classification divides each leaflet into three sections called scallops, based on 'pleats' between sections rather than distinct splits in the leaflet body. The middle scallop of the posterior leaflet is usually the largest. By convention, the scallop nearest the left atrial appendage is scallop 1, the central scallop 2 and the more medial scallop number 3. The posterior leaflet scallops are thus termed P1, P2 and P3, and face the corresponding A1, A2 and A3 scallops of the anterior leaflet (Fig. 1.11).

General anatomy and function

The leaflets are thin and mobile with a clear zone free of any attachments closest to the annulus, leading to a thickened rough zone on the ventricular side of the leaflet where chordae attach close to the line of coaptation. When the leaflets come together in systole, the chordae act like parachute cords and prevent the leaflets prolapsing back into the left atrium. They also help pull the coaptation zone together, with the leaflet tips pointing towards the LV apex, in line with the LV long axis. The line of coaptation does not normally extend beyond the level of the atrioventricular junction (see 📖 p.178).

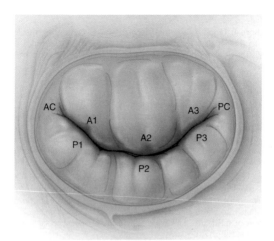

Fig. 1.11 The mitral valve viewed from the left atrium. The scallops of the anterior (A) and posterior (P) leaflets, and the anterolateral (AC) and postero-lateral commissure (PC) are labelled. Reproduced with permission from Verma S., Mesana T.G. (2009) Mitral-Valve Repair for Mitral-Valve Prolapse *NEJM*; 361: 2261–2269. Copyright 2009 Massachusetts Medical Society. All rights reserved.

Chordae

The chordae tendinae are thin fibrous strands connecting the leaflets either to the papillary muscles or directly to the infero-posterior wall of the LV. Chords from both papillary muscles insert into both mitral valve leaflets.

The chordae can be subdivided by their type and attachment:
- 1st order chordae—multiple thin chords attached to the free edge of the leaflets along the coaptation line
- 2nd order chordae—thicker structures attached to the mid portion of the leaflet body (usually in the rough zone)
- 3rd order chordae from the leaflet direct to the ventricular wall and only attached to the posterior leaflet—to reach the anterior leaflet they would have to cross either the inflow or outflow tract.

Stronger chordae running from the tips of the papillary muscles to the rough zone are termed *strut chordae* and are prominent on imaging. The arrangement and number of chordae inserting into each portion of the leaflets may play a role in the development of leaflet prolapse, where a section of the leaflet falls back behind the atrioventricular junction in systole (see 📖 p.178).

Papillary muscles

The papillary muscles arise from the LV lateral wall and act as anchor points for chordae, in addition to providing dynamic tension on the chordae and leaflets during the cardiac cycle. Typically, *posteromedial* and *anterolateral* papillary muscles are described (Fig. 1.12) but these are often groups of muscle bundles rather than single entities. The bases of these papillary groups may be connected by bridging bundles. The anterolateral papillary muscle is usually larger and derives its blood supply from the circumflex artery or a diagonal branch of the left anterior descending artery. The posteromedial papillary muscle often has multiple muscle heads and derives its blood supply from the posterior descending artery (which most commonly arises from the right coronary artery). It is more prone to ischaemic rupture than the anterolateral papillary muscle.

Left ventricular wall

The wall of the LV to which the papillary muscles attach is also important, providing anchorage for the papillary muscles and facilitating correct alignment of the chordae with the valve. Normal systolic contraction reduces both the short and long axis dimensions of the LV cavity and maintains the correct alignment and distance between the papillary muscles and valve leaflets. Along with papillary muscle contraction, this is vital as the fibrous chordae are fixed in length. A wall motion abnormality in the region of either papillary muscle will disrupt this arrangement, typically causing excess traction and systolic displacement of the leaflet into the LV cavity leading to failure of coaptation and 'functional' regurgitation (Fig. 1.13 and see 📖 p.182).

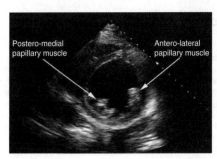

Fig. 1.12 Transthoracic image of the LV short axis demonstrating two papillary muscle groups. Although both are in the posterior portion of the cavity, the lateral muscle is relatively more anterior and termed the anterolateral papillary muscle.

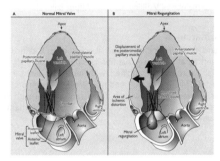

Fig. 1.13 Displacement of the ventricular wall and papillary muscle can lead to significant MR. Reproduced with permission from Levine R.A. Dynamic Mitral Regurgitation—More Than Meets the Eye *NEJM* 2004; 351:1681–1684. Copyright 2004 Massachusetts Medical Society. All rights reserved.

Normal mitral valve physiology

Diastole

The normal mitral valve opens widely in diastole allowing free passage of blood into the LV. The orifice is large, allowing flow despite the low pressure gradient from the left atrium to the LV.

Systole

The leaflets close and the thickened edges of the leaflet tips meet to form a tight seal. The papillary muscles and chordae apply tension to the leaflet body and tips, preventing the high pressure in the LV cavity forcing the leaflets into the left atrium.

- Mitral valve area   4–6cm^2
- Mitral annulus diameter in diastole   2.7 +/– 0.4cm
- Mitral annulus diameter in systole   2.9 +/– 0.3cm

Physiology of mitral stenosis

Effect on the left atrium

The normal mitral valve has an orifice area of 4–6cm^2 allowing unrestricted diastolic blood flow from the left atrium to the LV with no gradient between the two chambers. In MS, a pressure gradient develops. The left atrium adapts with hypertrophy and dilation and atrial contraction initially increases to maintain adequate LV filling.

While adequate trans-mitral flow may be maintained at rest, this is not the case during increased heart rate as diastole is shorter. Patients may therefore develop symptoms during exercise or other conditions, such as pregnancy.

Pulmonary pressure

Chronically-elevated pulmonary venous pressure leads to pulmonary hypertension and secondary effects on the right ventricle (RV). As the left atrium fails to maintain LV filling, cardiac output falls with resultant heart failure.

Atrial fibrillation

Restoring and maintaining effective atrial contraction is difficult in severe MS due to left atrial dilation. Atrial fibrillation is common. Unfortunately, loss of atrial contraction combined with increased heart rate further reduces diastolic filling of the LV and may precipitate symptoms (breathlessness) or worsening heart failure. Strict rate control with β-blockade or digoxin is required, and cardioversion or even ablation therapy may be needed in some patients.

General aspects of therapy

- Diuretic therapy to reduce pulmonary congestion improves symptoms.
- Excessive use can reduce LV filling and worsen peripheral perfusion.
- Prolonging diastole is helpful and rate limiting drugs, such as β blockers, calcium channel antagonists and digoxin, can be used.

Physiology of mitral regurgitation

Response of the ventricle

As in AR, the primary challenge to the LV is volume loading. In contrast to AR however, LV afterload is reduced as the stroke volume flows partially to the left atrium, a low pressure chamber. Consequently, the principal adaptive response in MR is LV dilation. A long period of dilation with preserved systolic function is typical, although the true contractile function of the ventricle can deteriorate significantly over time with no apparent change in systolic function due to the favourable reduction in afterload. The normal ventricle should be *hyperdynamic* with a high normal or supranormal ejection fraction. This explains the relatively high ejection fraction threshold of 60% when intervention is considered (see 📖 p.206).

As the LV dilates and becomes more spherical, altered papillary muscle and annular geometry may exacerbate progression to symptoms. Atrial fibrillation may also provoke decline although the effect is less marked than in MS.

General aspects of therapy

Arterial vasodilators may have less effect since afterload is not increased.

Effective medical therapy will depend on a number of factors:

Aetiology—intrinsic mitral valve disease or functional regurgitation?

If MR is secondary to LV dilation/adverse remodelling (i.e. functional regurgitation), both afterload reduction (arterial vasodilators) and preload reduction (venodilators, diuretics) may improve LV geometry and reduce the degree of regurgitation.

Fixed or dynamic regurgitant lesion

In fixed lesions (such as in rheumatic valvular heart disease), reducing preload will have no effect on the regurgitation but may improve symptoms by reducing pulmonary congestion.

Mitral valve prolapse

Prolapse can be worsened by reducing preload, as reduction in annulus size and fall in left atrial pressure exacerbate leaflet prolapse.

Hypertrophic cardiomyopathy

MR may be secondary to systolic anterior motion of the mitral valve and worsens if preload is reduced with diuretics or veno-dilators. Maintaining good hydration is important. β-blockers may be helpful to slow LV ejection and reduce the dynamic outflow tract gradient responsible for the effects on the mitral valve.

Acute mitral regurgitation
- The rapid rise in left atrial pressure and elevated LV end-diastolic pressure quickly lead to pulmonary oedema.
- Compensatory remodelling has not had time to occur and medical therapy has a limited role.

▶ Vasodilation and insertion of an intra-aortic balloon pump can be used as a bridge to definitive intervention (surgery).

Mixed mitral valve disease

As in AS, the pathophysiology and clinical findings are dependent on the dominant lesion:
- Dilated ventricle suggests dominant MR.
- Normal LV volume suggests dominant MS.

Both lesions will cause a dilated left atrium and frequently lead to atrial fibrillation.

High trans-mitral velocities will occur in significant MR with potential overestimation of the degree of MS. Multiple assessment techniques (including direct orifice planimetry) are required to ensure correct assessment.

In complex mixed mitral valve disease the use of a dynamic study may be revealing. Exercise echocardiography is easily performed and can be used to assess both MS and MR during exertion.

Exercise during cardiac catheterisation is feasible but more challenging; it may still be required in selected cases.

Management is determined by the dominant lesion although the threshold for intervention may be lower given the combined stress on the left atrium and ventricle.

Tricuspid valve anatomy

The inflow valve between the right atrium and RV is the largest cardiac valve and more apical than the corresponding plane of the mitral valve (Fig. 1.14). The tricuspid valve has similarly complex components as the mitral valve, though the pressures it has to resist are lower. The very low right atrial pressure explains the need for a large diastolic opening area.

Components of the valve complex:
• Tricuspid annulus
• Valve leaflets
• Chordae tendinae
• Papillary muscles
• RV

Tricuspid annulus

The annulus of the tricuspid valve is larger than that of the mitral valve but similarly shaped, being curved along one side and relatively flat along the other. It is less fibrous than the mitral annulus as there is no connection to the central fibrous body.

Valve leaflets

The valve has three leaflets, separated by indentations rather than true divisions with commissures (Fig. 1.15):
• Anterior/anterolateral leaflet—the largest
• Septal leaflet—with most support from the right fibrous trigone
• Posterior leaflet—usually the smallest.

The relative size of the leaflets is variable and small additional leaflets are occasionally present.

Adjacent structures

The ostium of the coronary sinus and the atrioventricular node lie close to the septal leaflet and can be damaged during tricuspid valve intervention.

Chordae tendinae

Each leaflet has chordae running to each papillary muscle, in the same fashion as the mitral valve. These can also be subdivided into first, second and third order chordae according to their origin and point of insertion. There are also slightly different fan-shaped chordae running from muscle heads to the free edge of the leaflets, with additional chords running deep to the free zone and attaching to the leaflet base.

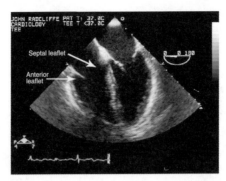

Fig. 1.14 Transoesophageal echocardiography demonstrating the anterior and septal leaflets of the tricuspid valve. Note the apical displacement of the tricuspid valve relative to the mitral valve.

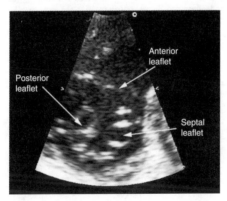

Fig. 1.15 Transthoracic short axis image zoomed in to the tricuspid valve demonstrating the three separate leaflets.

Right ventricle

The RV muscle ensures correct alignment of the papillary muscles to the valve leaflets. Dilation of the ventricle leads to displacement of the papillary muscles, preventing accurate coaptation and further distortion of the annulus, both of which can result in TR (Fig. 1.16). RV dilation typically displaces the anterior and posterior leaflets as the sepal leaflet connects to the relatively fibrous portion of the annulus.

Normal tricuspid valve physiology

Diastole

The low pressure gradient between the right atrium and RV requires a large size of the open tricuspid valve to ensure free passage of blood (driven principally by the central venous pressure) into the right heart.

Systole

The leaflets close and the thickened edges of the leaflet tips meet to form a tight seal. The papillary muscles and chordae apply tension to the leaflet body and tips, preventing increased pressure in the RV cavity forcing the leaflets into the right atrium.

- Tricuspid valve area   7–8cm^2
- Tricuspid annulus diameter   2.7–2.9cm

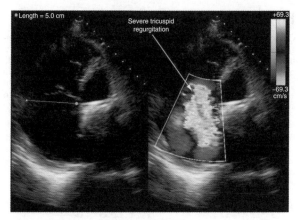

Fig. 1.16 Transthoracic echocardiogram demonstrating a severely dilated right ventricle with tricuspid regurgitation due to dilation of the tricuspid annulus. See also Plate 1.

Physiology of tricuspid stenosis

Obstruction of the tricuspid valve is rare, and usually rheumatic or congenital in origin. Other causes include carcinoid syndrome and a prosthetic tricuspid valve. The effects on the right heart mirror those of MS on the left heart. However, since the right heart is a low pressure system even a small gradient across the tricuspid valve is sufficient to elevate right atrial pressure. For example, a pressure gradient of 5mmHg is enough to cause symptoms and signs of right atrial hypertension.

Effect on the right atrium

Right atrial hypertrophy and dilation develop to maintain RV filling, with increased dependence on atrial contraction. As the atrium fails or atrial arrhythmia intervenes, RV preload and cardiac output fall (initially during exercise but eventually at rest).

Physiology of tricuspid regurgitation

Response of the ventricle

The haemodynamic effects of tricuspid regurgitation (TR) on the RV are similar to those of MR on the LV. Volume loading leads to progressive dilation, albeit with a number of differences:

The tricuspid annulus

The reduced fibrous support for the tricuspid valve annulus may lead to earlier dilation and worsening TR in response to RV dilation, creating a vicious circle.

Effect on the left ventricle

As TR progresses, the RV and right atrium dilate further and RV systolic failure ensues. Elevated RV end-diastolic pressure and paradoxical septal motion in turn reduce LV function. Elevated left-sided pressures lead to increased pulmonary pressure and further exacerbation of right heart failure.

Pulmonary pressures

The degree of pulmonary hypertension and its potential reversibility are vital to the successful treatment of TR with RV failure: if the RV afterload cannot be reduced then the likelihood of significant improvement in RV function is low.

Acute tricuspid regurgitation

- Acute TR is rare but can complicate RV infarction, particularly if the papillary muscles are involved.
- A sudden elevation in venous pressure leads to hepatic congestion and severe hepatic necrosis can develop.
- Peripheral oedema, systemic hypotension, and elevated venous pressure are the clinical clues in this scenario.

▶ Management is challenging—diuresis to relieve oedema needs to be balanced with the need to maintain RV filling pressure. Inotropes to augment RV function can be useful.

Pulmonary valve anatomy

This trileaflet valve prevents regurgitation of blood from the pulmonary artery to the RV and is very similar in size and morphology to the aortic valve. There are, however, some important differences:
- Thinner valve leaflets
- No coronary ostia and no discrete sinuses
- Muscular annulus.

The pulmonary valve complex consists of:
- RV outflow tract
- Semilunar valve leaflets
- Interleaflet triangles
- Pulmonary annulus.

Right ventricular outflow tract (the infundibulum)

The RV outflow tract is a free standing 'sleeve' arising from the RV, just beyond the supraventricular crest—a prominent muscle band in the RV. It is a muscular smooth-walled funnel leading to the pulmonary valve, and termed the *infundibulum*. Contraction in systole is significant, though without RV outflow tract obstruction.

Semilunar valve leaflets

The pulmonary valve consists of three symmetrical hemispherical (semilunar) leaflets which are slightly thinner than the aortic valve leaflets (Fig. 1.17).
- Anterior leaflet
- Right leaflet
- Left leaflet.

Interleaflet triangles ('trigones')

The attachments of the valve leaflets are semi-circular, leading to triangular interleaflet areas between the apices of the points of insertion to the pulmonary arterial wall. These regions are important surgical landmarks, particularly if enlargement of the outflow tract and annulus is required.

Pulmonary annulus

There is no true circular annulus supporting the pulmonary valve. Since the attachments to the pulmonary trunk are semilunar, the 'annulus' is coronet shaped.

In contrast to the aortic valve, the surrounding tissue is exclusively muscular with little fibrous tissue. Since the pulmonary valve is separated from the RV inflow by the infundibulum, there is no continuity with the tricuspid valve.

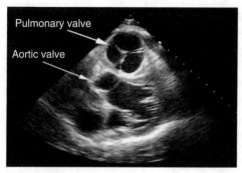

Fig. 1.17 In this patient with severe pulmonary arterial dilation, unusually clear views of the pulmonary valve could be obtained on transthoracic echocardiography.

Physiology of pulmonary stenosis

Obstruction of RV outflow can be sub-valvular, valvular or supra-valvular and may occur as an isolated lesion or in combination with complex congenital heart disease. The exact effects of the stenotic lesion are dependent on the site of obstruction, compliance of the RV and the presence of any additional cardiac lesions.

Effect on the right ventricle

• The development of a pressure gradient between the RV and pulmonary artery leads to ventricular hypertrophy to increase systolic pressure. This is maintained until the RV starts to fail or the effect of other cardiac disease supervenes.
• Secondary hypertrophy of the RV may include the muscular infundibulum below the valve, leading to further outflow obstruction.
• The elevated RV pressure is transmitted to the right atrium. If there is a shunt at the ventricular or atrial level (or a patent foramen ovale) then right to left shunting with consequent cyanosis may develop.
• The response of the RV is also dependent on the timing of lesion development. Structural stenosis present in the neonate leads to myocyte hyperplasia and an increased capillary network, whereas stenosis developing in the mature heart leads to myocyte hypertrophy with no effect on vascular development.

Physiology of pulmonary regurgitation

While the pathophysiology of pulmonary regurgitation (PR) is broadly similar to AR, there are important differences. Both lesions can be well tolerated for many years:

Pulmonary pressure

• The pulmonary circulation has relatively low resistance compared to the systemic vasculature and flow into the pulmonary vascular bed requires less work.
• The RV can act as a simple conduit for forward flow into the pulmonary artery, relying on systemic venous return and right atrial contraction (as typified by with Fontan circulation). Forward flow can often be maintained, even significant PR.
• Conditions which raise pulmonary vascular resistance exacerbate PR.

Response of the ventricle

▶ As with AR, RV volume overload leads to dilation. The compliance of the RV, affected by fibrosis and hypertrophy, is central to the adaptive response and ability to maintain normal RV wall stress.

General aspects of therapy

- Appropriate medical therapy depends on the constellation of lesions and their secondary effects—reducing congestion with diuretics and preventing arrhythmia are important.
- RV dysfunction may complicate management and require support with inotropes.

Assessment of valvular heart disease

Introduction

The assessment of a patient with known or suspected valvular heart disease requires careful integration of information and data derived from:
- Background clinical information
- History and description of symptoms
- Clinical examination
- Electrocardiogram (ECG) and chest X-ray
- Echocardiography
- Other imaging/investigations.

In many patients this is sufficient to guide medical therapy and appropriate follow up arrangements. Additional data may be required for some to further clarify the aetiology, severity and effects of the valvular heart disease. Patients with acute severe manifestations of valvular heart disease often present in crisis and require immediate assessment whilst stabilisation is achieved. Often the diagnosis is confirmed while arrangements for definitive intervention (e.g. surgery) are being made.

The importance of symptoms

The management of many patients depends on whether symptoms can be attributed to the effects of the valve lesion. It is important to ensure that adequate time and credence are placed on the patient's description of their current functional state and how this has changed with time, before moving on to detailed imaging studies.

Clinical evaluation

Clinical evaluation often begins before meeting the patient, usually via information from the clinical record or referring physician. This may include important details on co-morbidity, current medical therapy, social circumstances and the patient's expectations.

History

The clinical encounter with the patient should focus on a careful detailed history, paying specific attention to the following:
- Reason for referral—incidental murmur or symptoms?
- Onset and progression of symptoms
- Previous treatment and its effect(s)
- Risk factors for cardiac disease: rheumatic fever, ischaemic heart disease?
- Co-morbidities
- Social circumstances and quality of life
- Patient expectations and understanding.

Symptoms

More detail of the symptoms caused by each valve lesion is discussed in later chapters, but some are common to all valvular heart disease often due to the deleterious effects on cardiac efficiency:

- Breathlessness—usually on effort unless severe heart failure is present
- Fatigue—due to reduced forward stroke volume and perfusion
- Orthopnoea—if pulmonary oedema is present
- Peripheral oedema—in significant right heart disease
- Angina—can occur without underlying coronary artery disease, particularly in AS
- Syncope—in lesions causing fixed cardiac output (AS and MS)
- Palpitations—often due to atrial fibrillation.

Typically, these symptoms are vague and have insidious onset. Patients, particularly the elderly, may not have recognised a specific symptom and instead reduced their daily workload. Careful questioning to compare their current level of activity with the year before can be useful to characterize the speed and extent of decline.

If doubt over a patient's current functional capacity remains then discussion with the patient's family and primary care physician may prove helpful.

Current treatment

Many patients may have already received medical therapy appropriate for their valvular heart disease either as primary treatment or as coincidental therapy for pre-existing cardiac disease, e.g. hypertension. Clarifying when the patient started these treatments (a diuretic for example) and how this has affected them can aid in the overall evaluation and likelihood of improvement with further medical therapy.

Co-morbidities

A full clinical history will include details of prior and current medical conditions. In anticipation of future surgical intervention, the details of specific co-morbid conditions should be sought:

- Diabetes—coronary artery disease?
- Pulmonary disease—long term bronchodilator/home oxygen therapy?
- Arteriopathy—claudication or transient ischaemic attack?
- Neurological disease—limitation of mobility, cognitive impairment?
- Renal impairment—stable or progressive?
- Body mass index—wound healing issues?
- Thrombosis/bleeding problems—may affect choice of prosthesis.

Social circumstances and quality of life

The key questions here are:
- What will intervention achieve?
- Are symptoms intrusive?
- Is surgical intervention appropriate?
- Will the patient retain / regain an independent existence?
- Patient motivation—do they wish to undergo invasive assessment or treatment?

Involvement of family members may be useful when discussing potential intervention, particularly in very elderly patients.

Patient expectations

Patients have an increasingly good understanding of the problem and potential treatment options due to the wealth of easily accessible medical information. However, it remains important for the clinician to explore what patients understand about their heart disease, and how treatments may help.

Some patients may decline intervention based on a misunderstanding of the risks and complications, or base their judgement on experience of a relative or friend. Conversely, they may have unrealistic expectations of what is available or appropriate. The clinician must ensure that a patient's choice is based on the correct information and balance of risk and benefit.

Clinical examination

A full and systematic examination should be performed to identify any valve or other cardiac pathology and evidence of haemodynamic decompensation (principally heart failure). Additional systems should be examined as directed by information from the clinical history.

Attention should be paid to the following:
- General body habitus
- Dentition—risk of IE
- Pulse character, rhythm and volume
- Blood pressure
- Venous pressure
- Apex beat position and character
- 1st and 2nd heart sounds
- Murmurs (including accentuation manoeuvres)
- 3rd or 4th heart sounds
- Lung bases—crackles or effusions
- Sacral oedema
- Peripheral oedema
- Peripheral pulses.

Electrocardiogram and chest X-ray

The ECG and chest X-ray add additional useful information to support the diagnosis and are part of the overall cardiac assessment.

The ECG should be assessed for:
- Rhythm—sinus rhythm or atrial fibrillation?
- Tachycardia—may reflect decompensation
- Cardiac axis—ischaemia or hypertrophy?
- Conduction system—additional sino-atrial disease or atrioventricular block?
- P wave morphology—may suggest atrial enlargement
- LV hypertrophy—may reflect pressure overload
- Bundle branches—heart failure with left bundle branch block?
- Ischaemia—evidence of recent infarction?

The chest X-ray provides information on:
- Cardiac size
- Shape of cardiac silhouette—atrial enlargement?
- Pulmonary congestion
- Pleural effusions
- Pulmonary hypertension
- Aortic dilation
- Additional pulmonary pathology.

Brief guide to the most common murmurs

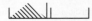

Aortic stenosis
see 📖 p.100

Harsh, rasping, sometimes musical ejection murmur
Upper right sternal edge, radiating to carotids
Slow rising pulse, soft/absent A_2

Aortic regurgitation
see 📖 p.132

Early diastolic de-crescendo murmur
(± systolic flow murmur)
Lower left sternal edge
Collapsing pulse, displaced hyperdynamic apex

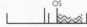

Mitral regurgitation
see 📖 p.190

Soft, blowing, monotonous pansystolic murmur
Apex, radiating to axilla
Displaced, hyperdynamic apex

Mitral stenosis
see 📖 p.156

Low-pitched, quiet mid-diastolic rumble
Apex, no radiation
Opening snap, 'tapping' apex, loud P_2

Grading of systolic murmurs (Levine, 1933)

1 Barely audible
2 Soft but readily detected
3 Prominent
4 Loud, usually with thrill
5 Very loud with thrill
6 So loud, can be heard with the stethoscope just off the chest

How to recognize an innocent ('flow') murmur

- Soft ejection systolic murmur
- Grade ≤ 2
- Usually heard along left sternal edge, occasionally at the apex
- Normal heart sounds
- No associated thrills or added sounds
- No signs of LV dilation
- Normal ECG and chest X-ray

▶ Echocardiography is not required for an innocent murmur
▶ Diastolic, pansystolic and loud murmurs (grade 4+) are seldom 'innocent'

Transthoracic echocardiography

Cardiac ultrasound (echocardiography) is the investigation of choice for patients with suspected valvular heart disease and can provide detailed data:

- Valve morphology
- Type of valvular heart disease
- Aetiology of valvular lesion
- Severity of valvular lesion
- Secondary effects of valvular lesion
- Cardiac structure and function
- Chamber size
- Great vessel anatomy
- Additional cardiac pathology.

Echocardiography is appropriate for any patient in whom the clinical picture suggests valve dysfunction. This includes unexplained breathlessness or syncope with signs of valvular heart disease, or deterioration of pre-existing disease. New or worsening clinical heart failure warrants echocardiography to exclude both valvular and non-valvular causes.

Severely unwell patients with suspected acute valve dysfunction need immediate echocardiography. For presentations over days/weeks, the echocardiogram can usually wait 24–72 hours, depending on the clinical status of the patient.

A full description of a standard transthoracic echocardiogram is beyond the scope of this chapter. A summary is presented to assist focused assessment of a valve lesion.

Transthoracic echocardiography: valve anatomy

Parasternal views

The starting point for a transthoracic echocardiographic examination is the parasternal window, with the probe placed in the upper left parasternal position between the ribs and manipulated to visualize the heart in both long and short axis. Medial angulation allows visualization of the RV.

Parasternal long axis view (Fig. 2.1)

- Aortic valve—non-coronary and right-coronary cusp
- Aortic root—sinuses and sinotubular junction
- Mitral valve—A1/2 and P2/3

Right ventricular inflow view (Fig. 2.2)

- Tricuspid valve—septal and anterior leaflets
- Coronary sinus and inferior vena cava

Parasternal short axis view (Fig. 2.3)

- Aortic valve—all three leaflets and coronary ostia
- Mitral valve—all six segments
- Tricuspid valve—septal and anterior leaflets
- Pulmonary valve—anterior and right leaflets

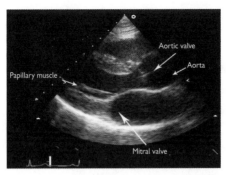

Fig. 2.1 Parasternal long axis view.

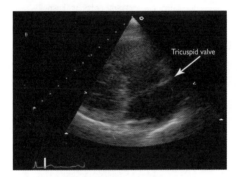

Fig. 2.2 Right ventricular inflow view.

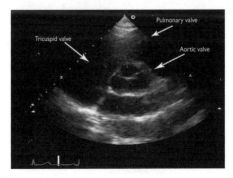

Fig. 2.3 Parasternal short axis view.

Apical views

The probe is placed over the cardiac apex to visualise all four chambers. Anterior angulation will bring the LV outflow tract (the '5th' chamber) into view.

Apical 4-chamber (Fig. 2.4)
- Mitral valve—A2/3 and P1/2 segments
- Tricuspid valve—septal and anterior or posterior leaflets

Apical 5-chamber (Fig. 2.5)
- Aortic valve—right-coronary and non-coronary leaflets

Apical 2-chamber (Fig. 2.6)
- Mitral valve—anterior leaflet en-face

Apical 3-chamber
- Mitral valve—A1/2 and P2/3 segments.
- Aortic valve—non-coronary and right coronary cusp

(Effectively the parasternal long axis view rotated through 90°)

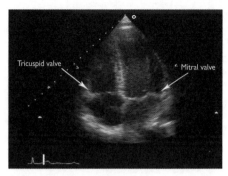

Fig. 2.4 Apical 4-chamber view.

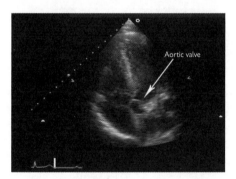

Fig. 2.5 Apical 5-chamber view.

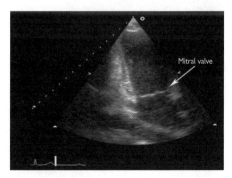

Fig. 2.6 Apical 2-chamber view.

Subcostal views

The probe is placed on the epigastrium and directed below the ribs to image the heart through the diaphragm.

Subcostal long axis (Fig. 2.7)

- Tricuspid valve—septal and lateral leaflets
- Mitral valve—A2/3 and P2/3 segments

Subcostal short axis (Fig. 2.8)

- Aortic valve—all three leaflets
- Mitral valve—all six segments
- Pulmonary valve—variable view

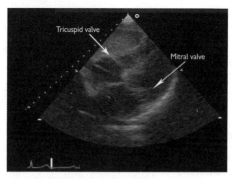

Fig. 2.7 Subcostal long axis view.

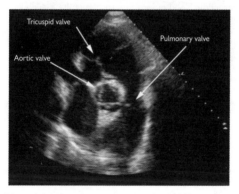

Fig. 2.8 Subcostal short axis view.

Assessment of valve function with echocardiography

All valves are routinely assessed in a standard study using the following modalities:
- Colour flow mapping
- Continuous wave Doppler
- Pulse wave Doppler.

If a valve lesion is detected then further quantification may be undertaken. Depending on the lesion this may include:
- Pressure half time
- Continuity equation
- Measurement of vena contracta
- Proximal isovelocity surface area (PISA)
- Regurgitant fraction.

Colour flow mapping

Colour pulse wave Doppler imaging is used to interrogate an area of blood flow. The direction and velocity of flow is colour-coded and super-imposed over the 2D greyscale image.

By convention, blood moving towards the probe is encoded in shades of red and blood moving away from the probe in shades of blue (Fig. 2.9). Blood moving faster than the limit of velocity detection (the Nyquist limit) appears in the colours of the opposite end of the spectrum 'aliasing'.

Limitations

While providing a visual demonstration of blood flow, it is important to understand the limitations of this modality for assessment of the severity of a valve lesion:
- Aliasing can occur at a velocity as low as 0.75m/s and is dependent on image depth and probe frequency
- Frame rates are reduced compared to plain 2D imaging
- Machine settings can drastically alter the appearance, particularly the colour scale setting
- The accuracy of the Doppler signal is most accurate for flow in line with the beam—more than 30° of angulation leads to significant error
- The colour will depend on the direction of flow relevant to the probe and the alignment angles effect on measured velocity.

Colour flow should only be used as an initial assessment of valvular flow. Additional methods of quantification are always used to avoid significant over- or under-estimation.

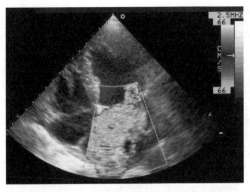

Fig. 2.9 Colour flow mapping of MR. Note the large 'blue flame' of regurgitation.
See also **Plate 2**.

Continuous wave Doppler

By transmitting and receiving along a single line of interrogation, continuous wave Doppler presents a visual display of all detected velocities along that line against time (Fig. 2.10). The spectral display shows blood moving towards the transducer as signals above the baseline and blood moving away below the baseline. The density of the signal represents the proportion of blood flow at that velocity. Mean and peak velocities can be measured, allowing estimation of mean and peak pressure drop.

Limitations

In practical terms, continuous wave Doppler can detect flow at any velocity, but there are important limitations:
- All velocities along the sample line are detected. Precise localization is not possible and can lead to misidentification of signals (e.g. MR can be mistaken for AS)
- The alignment of the signal with flow is important for accuracy—misalignment >15–30° introduces significant error
- The true peak velocity will only be measured if it is in the line of interrogation—alignment should be confirmed in multiple planes

The simplified Bernoulli equation can be used to convert peak velocity to a peak pressure drop:

Pressure drop = 4 × peak velocity²

Pulse wave Doppler

In order to localize the signal of interest along the line of interrogation, a pulse of Doppler can be transmitted and then received. The required time interval defines the position of the sample volume on the 2D image. This technique allows precise measurement in specific sites, e.g. the LV outflow tract. The pulsed wave signal is displayed in the same manner as continuous wave Doppler (Fig. 2.11).

Limitations

- Aliasing occurs at a set velocity dependent on the depth of sampling and probe frequency.
- Blood moving faster than the Nyquist limit is not correctly encoded according to direction and speed and 'wraps around' the baseline.
- The angle of interrogation has an impact on the accuracy of velocity encoding.

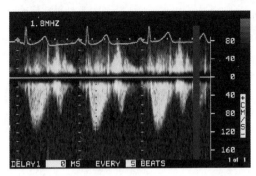

Fig. 2.10 Continuous wave Doppler through the LV outflow tract and aortic valve demonstrating normal outflow velocity signal.

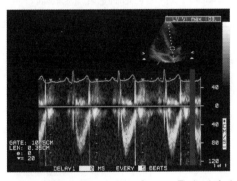

Fig. 2.11 Pulsed wave Doppler from the LV outflow tract. The band of velocities is narrow indicating smooth laminar flow.

Pressure half time

The pressure half time (P½t) a measure of low velocity flow, is the time taken for the measured pressure drop across a valve to fall to half its initial value (Fig. 2.12). The smaller the valve area (higher degree of stenosis), the longer it takes for blood to pass through and the longer the pressure half time. P½t is inversely proportional to valve area, which can be calculated with certain assumptions.

It is most commonly applied in MS:

Mitral valve area = 220/Pressure half time

Limitations

- The deceleration slope can be curved making accurate measurement difficult—use of the mid diastolic slope is advised.
- LV filling is dependent on left atrial compliance and LV diastolic function and may vary significantly. Poor LV relaxation will elevate P½t. This may be relevant in the elderly or those with degenerative calcific MS in whom LV fibrosis and delayed relaxation are common.
- P½t does not accurately reflect changes in valve area during intervention e.g. balloon valvuloplasty.
- P½t is underestimated in patients with significant AR, in whom LV diastolic pressure rises rapidly.

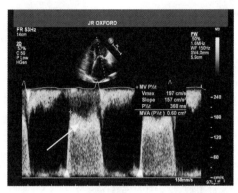

Fig. 2.12 Spectral Doppler of mitral valve inflow. Measurement of the deceleration slope from the peak of the mitral E-wave (dashed line, arrowed) allows calculation of P½t and valve area.

Continuity equation

The measurement of valve area in AS is the prime use for this technique, which is based on the principle that all blood within the LV outflow tract (LVOT) crosses the aortic valve (AV) (Fig. 2.13).

> LVOT flow = aortic valve flow

Flow is the product of cross sectional area and velocity, therefore:

> LVOT area × LVOT velocity = AV area × AV velocity

Therefore:

> AV area = LVOT area × LVOT velocity/AV velocity

The LVOT cross sectional area can be measured using a short axis view or by measuring its diameter in the parasternal long axis view and deriving the area by assuming a circular shape. LVOT velocity is measured using pulse wave Doppler and aortic valve velocity using continuous wave Doppler.

Either the peak velocity or velocity time integral (VTI; a summation of all the velocities) can be used.

Limitations

- Deriving the LVOT area involves squaring its radius (half the diameter) so any measurement error is magnified.
- LVOT velocity may not be uniform e.g. in sub-aortic stenosis.
- The measurement derived is smaller than the anatomical valve area due to contraction of flow above the valve orifice.
- The valve area may be significantly underestimated if stroke volume is reduced due to LV failure.

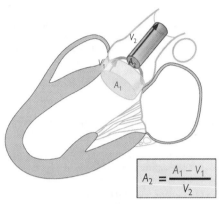

$$A_2 = \frac{A_1 - V_1}{V_2}$$

Fig. 2.13 Schematic diagram of the continuity equation. A_1 and V_1 are the left ventricular outflow tract area and velocity, A_2 and V_2 the aortic valve area and velocity Reproduced with permission from Baumgartner H., Hung J, Bermejo J. *et al.* Echocardiographic assessment of valve stenosis: EAE/ASE recommendations for clinical practice. *European Journal of Echocardiography* 2009; 10:1–25, Oxford University Press.

Vena contracta

The neck of a flow jet as it passes through a narrowed valve orifice is the vena contracta (Fig. 2.14). It usually consists of laminar flow at high velocity with a diameter slightly smaller than the anatomical orifice.

The size of the vena contracta is unaltered by pressure or flow, making it a reliable indicator of orifice area.

Assessment of the vena contracta is most helpful in regurgitant lesions (primarily AR and MR).

Limitations

- A small width is measured (usually <1cm)—accuracy may be difficult.
- The regurgitant orifice may vary in size leading to a variable vena contracta.
- Changes in colour flow settings alter the appearance of the jet.
- Eccentric jets flatten against walls and become elliptical in cross-sectional profile, increasing the error of measurement.

Proximal isovelocity surface area (PISA)

Blood accelerates towards an orifice and this occurs in roughly hemispheric shells of flow with higher velocity and decreasing surface area. By adjusting the settings of colour flow mapping these hemispheres can be identified (Fig. 2.15).

The effective regurgitant orifice area (EROA) can be derived by measuring the radius of the hemisphere (r) at that velocity (Va) if the peak regurgitant velocity is also known (PeakV):

$$EROA = (2\pi r^2 \times Va)/PeakV$$

This method is only robust for central jets that allow good alignment with the Doppler signal—the usual application is in MR with a central jet. Assessment of eccentric jets is usually inaccurate.

Most modern echocardiography platforms are able to perform semi-automated calculation of EROA once the PISA radius has been measured.

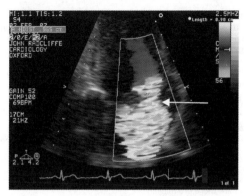

Fig. 2.14 Zoomed view of MR using colour flow mapping to demonstrate the vena contracta (arrowed). See also **Plate 3**.

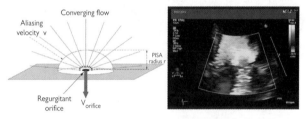

Fig. 2.15 The left hand panel is a schematic representation of PISA measurement. The right hand panel is a colour flow image showing the hemispheric 'shell' of flow convergence. The colour scale baseline has been altered so that a clear hemisphere of flow at a single velocity is seen, identified by transition of the colour jet (from blue to yellow, arrowed) at the limit of the velocity range.
Left hand panel reproduced from Irvine T., Li XK, Sahn D.J., Kenny A. (2002) Assessment of mitral regurgitation *Heart*; 88:11–19 with permission from BMJ Publishing Group Ltd. See also **Plate 4**.

Regurgitant fraction

The volume of regurgitation through a valve can be expressed as an absolute volume or as a proportion of the stroke volume (regurgitant fraction). This can be calculated using echocardiography in two different ways:
- Derived from the EROA
- By comparing stroke volume at two separate sites (the more common approach).

In MR, less blood will flow through the LVOT than through the mitral valve, and the difference between the two is the volume of regurgitation.

Limitations

The technique relies on significant assumptions and multiple measurements, each with scope for error.

Specific limitations include:
- Cross sectional area is derived by squaring the measured radius—errors are therefore magnified
- The mitral annulus is oval in shape and accurate assessment of cross sectional area is difficult
- Ensuring that the sites of velocity and cross sectional area measurement are the same is difficult
- Multiple valve lesions introduce error and invalidate the assumptions underlying this technique.

Assessment of left ventricular function

An important factor in the management of any patient with valvular heart disease is accurate quantification of LV function. Many patients attend for serial echocardiography and changing LV function may indicate the need for intervention.

Calculating ejection fraction

All patients should have their LV ejection fraction measured using the best available technique. The minimum acceptable measurement is Simpson's bi-plane method. Reliance on M-mode or 2D single plane measurement should be avoided.

The LV endocardial border is outlined in two orthogonal planes (usually the apical 4- and 2-chamber views) in end-diastole and end-systole. The software derives volumes and ejection fraction using complex modelling (Fig. 2.16).

Improving the assessment

- If the images limit accurate assessment, echocardiographic contrast should be given to opacify the LV and improve endocardial border definition.
- Advances in three-dimensional imaging allow even greater accuracy in LV volume measurement. This should be the method of choice if appropriate equipment and expertise are available.

Assessment of right ventricular function

Quantification of right ventricular function is more challenging due to the asymmetric shape of the right ventricle. Measurement of the excursion of the tricuspid annulus towards the apex during systole can be used to score right ventricular function. New techniques, including three-dimensional volumetric analysis, are in development.

Tricuspid annular plane systolic excursion (TAPSE)

An M-mode cursor is positioned at the base of the right ventricular free wall at the level of the tricuspid annulus and the amount of systolic excursion measured: (Fig. 2.17):

RV dysfunction	Normal	Mild	Moderate	Severe
TAPSE	16 – 20mm	11 – 15mm	6 – 10mm	<6mm

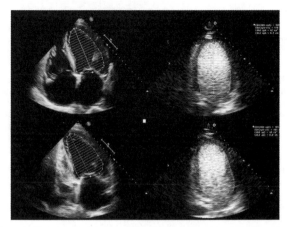

Fig. 2.16 The left hand panels demonstrate manual tracing of the ventricular cavity in diastole from the apical 4-chamber (top) and 2-chamber (bottom) views. The right hand panels demonstrate the same measurements in a patient with poor acoustic windows - contrast has been given to opacify the LV cavity.

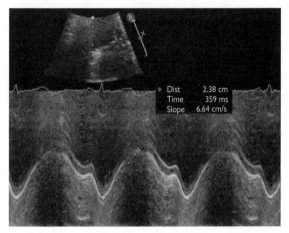

Fig. 2.17 Example of tricuspid annular plane systolic excursion (TAPSE) measurement via an M-mode cursor through the tricuspid annulus.

Assessment of pulmonary pressure

A full echocardiographic assessment of valvular heart disease should include RV size and function along with an estimation of pulmonary pressure.

Principle behind the calculation of systolic pressure

The RV ejects blood into the pulmonary arteries so RV systolic pressure equals that in the pulmonary arteries [in the absence of pulmonary stenosis (PS)]. RV systolic pressure can be estimated from tricuspid valve flow since the majority of tricuspid valves are not fully competent and regurgitant pressure across the valve is determined by the difference in pressure.

TR pressure = RV systolic pressure − RA pressure

Therefore:

RV (i.e. PA systolic) pressure = TR pressure + RA pressure

The peak TR pressure jet can be estimated from the peak velocity using the modified Bernoulli equation (Fig. 2.18):

$$PA\ systolic\ pressure = 4 \times (peak\ TR\ velocity)^2 + RA\ pressure$$

TR velocity can be measured using continuous wave Doppler and the RA pressure estimated from the jugular venous pressure (or quantified using the size of the inferior vena cava and degree of inspiratory collapse).

Diastolic pulmonary pressures

Similarly, the end velocity of a PR signal equates to the pulmonary artery *diastolic* pressure:

Regurgitant pressure = pulmonary pressure − diastolic RV pressure

PA diastolic pressure = regurgitant pressure + diastolic RV pressure

Using the Bernoulli equation for regurgitant pressure, and assuming RV end-diastolic pressure ~ RA pressure:

$$RV\ diastolic\ pressure = 4 \times (end\ PR\ velocity)^2 + RA\ pressure$$

In practice this assessment is rarely used.

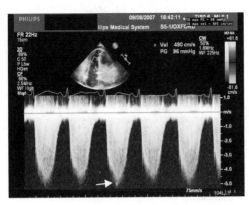

Fig. 2.18 Continuous wave Doppler of TR. The peak velocity of 5m/s (arrowed) suggests a peak pressure drop of 100mmHg indicating severe pulmonary hypertension. See also **Plate 5**.

Transoesophageal echocardiography

In the majority of patients, a transthoracic study is sufficient to confirm the diagnosis and guide further management; however transoesophageal imaging can be very useful in some scenarios:

- Limited quality transthoracic assessment
- Conflict of transthoracic assessment with clinical findings
- Complex mitral valve disease where surgery is contemplated
- Suspicion of IE
- Prosthetic valve dysfunction—in combination with transthoracic echocardiography
- Assessment of aortic root and ascending aorta.

The principles of assessment are the same as for transthoracic echocardiography, though the improved image quality increases the accuracy of measurements (Fig. 2.19).

Three-dimensional transoesophageal echocardiography

Newer platforms with real time 3D transoesophageal echocardiography are available and provide excellent imaging, particularly of the mitral valve (Fig. 2.20).

Initial experiences suggest this modality may be helpful in planning intervention and prior to/during mitral valve surgery, as the 3D image can be manipulated to replicate the 'surgeon's view' of the valve.

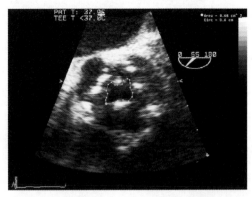

Fig. 2.19 Transoesophageal image showing a zoomed short axis view of the aortic valve in systole with direct planimetry of the aortic valve orifice (dotted line).

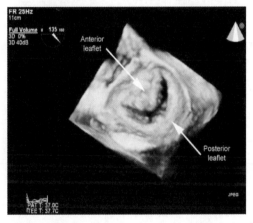

Fig. 2.20 Three-dimensional transoesophageal image of the mitral valve in early systole clearly demonstrating the anterior and posterior leaflets and atrial wall.

Selected normal values for echocardiography
Chamber sizes

Left ventricle	Septal thickness	0.6–1.2cm
	Diastolic dimensions	5.3cm (women) 5.9cm (men)
	Diastolic volume	104ml (women) 155ml (men)
	Systolic volume	49ml (women) 58ml (men)
	Ejection fraction (Simpson's bi-plane)	≥55%
	Mass	150g (women) 200g (men)
Left atrium	Long axis diameter (from 4-chamber view)	3.8cm (women) 4.0cm (men)
	Volume	52ml (women) 58ml (men)
Right ventricle	Basal diameter (from 4-chamber view)	2.8cm
	Base to apex length	7.9cm
Inferior vena cava	On inspiration	<1.5cm with collapse (RA pressure = 0–5)
Aortic root	Ascending aorta	2.1–3.4cm
	Aortic sinuses diameter	Correct to body surface area for most accurate assessment

Valve Doppler assessment

Aortic valve	Area	>2.0cm^2
	Peak velocity	<1.7m/s
	Annulus	1.4–2.6cm
	LVOT velocity	0.7–1.1m/s
Mitral valve	Pressure half time	40–70ms
	Valve area	4.0–6.0cm^2
	E velocity	0.6–1.3m/s
	A velocity	0.2–0.7m/s
	Deceleration slope	5.0 +/– 1.4m/s
	Annulus	2.7 +/– 0.4cm (diastole) 2.9 +/– 0.3cm (systole)
E/A ratio	Mitral inflow Doppler	1–2
Pulmonary valve	Pressure drop	<20mmHg
Tricuspid valve	Area	>7.0cm^2
	E velocity	0.3–0.7m/s
	Annulus	2.7–2.9cm

Stress testing

The use of a dynamic investigation to assess changes in cardiac perform-ance can be undertaken using a variety of techniques:
- Exercise electrocardiogram
- Exercise echocardiography
- Dobutamine stress echocardiography
- Exercise MUGA (multigated acquisition) scan using nuclear isotopes.

Exercise electrocardiogram

Patients frequently fail to recognize symptoms which cause limitation and instead attribute these changes to ageing or lack of fitness. Formal exercise testing can be useful to highlight poor exercise capacity and provide a baseline assessment of current functional status. Future repeat assessments can then highlight important changes.

The standard treadmill or bicycle ergometer stress test can be undertaken in patients with valvular heart disease to answer the following questions:
- Are symptoms such as dyspnoea and fatigue provoked at low workload in a patient who claims to be asymptomatic?
- Risk stratification in asymptomatic patients with AS (see below)
- Assessment of exercise capacity to facilitate advice regarding thresholds of exertion.

The ECG recorded during the stress test may be difficult to interpret due to changes secondary to LV hypertrophy—the routine use of an exercise ECG to assess for possible coronary artery disease is not recommended in this patient group.

Exercise testing is safe in the majority of patients with valvular heart disease but clinical judgement and appropriate supervision are required.

Contraindications
- Symptomatic severe AS
- Uncontrolled heart failure
- Unstable angina
- Unstable arrhythmia
- Acute myocarditis.

Risk stratification in aortic stenosis

Asymptomatic patients with significant AS (valve area $<1.2cm^2$) may be at risk of progression to symptoms and rapid decline.

Objective exercise testing for exertional symptoms may identify those patients in whom more rapid progression is likely.

80% of patients who demonstrate symptoms on exertion will develop spontaneous symptoms within 12 months. This may influence the timing of intervention.

Criteria for a positive exercise test in asymptomatic AS (standard Bruce protocol):
- Limiting dyspnoea, chest discomfort or dizziness
- ST depression >5mm
- >3 consecutive ventricular ectopics
- Fall in systolic blood pressure >20mmHg from baseline.

Exercise echocardiography

In patients with MR, assessment of regurgitation and LV function during exertion can be helpful. It is not uncommon for the assessment at rest to underestimate severity.

Dynamic changes in the mitral annulus and ischaemia affecting the ventricle and papillary muscles can lead to a rapid increase in the degree of MR. Further changes in LV ejection fraction and pulmonary pressure can also be assessed. A pulmonary arterial systolic pressure >60mmhg during exercise may be considered an indication for mitral valve surgery, even in asymptomatic MR.

Exercise echocardiography is practically challenging since images are required immediately after exercise. A dedicated supine bicycle couch allows simultaneous exercise and echocardiography.

Dobutamine stress echocardiography

Dobutamine stress echocardiography has poor sensitivity and specificity for the exclusion of ischaemic heart disease in patients with significant valvular heart disease and is not recommended in this setting.

It is particularly useful in the assessment of a patient with AS and poor LV function (see 📖 p.121) Low dose (up to 10mcg/kg/min) dobutamine stress echocardiography can address the following issues:

Functional reserve

- To determine if LV function improves, i.e. whether there is any functional reserve. If stroke volume increases by 20% or more, the surgical risk and long term outcome are considerably better (5% operative mortality compared to 32% in those where LV function does not improve).

Valve opening and gradient

- If valve area increases significantly with dobutamine, this suggests less severe valve disease and a primary problem with LV function.
- An increase in mean pressure drop to >30mmHg is suggestive of severe AS.

Dobutamine stress echocardiography in mitral stenosis

If there is discordance between the severity of MS with resting echocardiography and the degree of symptoms, a dobutamine stress echocardiogram can be used to identify exertion-induced pulmonary hypertension. Reduced atrial and ventricular compliance can lead to significant pulmonary hypertension with elevated heart rates, even in apparently moderate MS.

Criteria for a positive dobutamine stress echocardiogram in MS:
- Mean transmitral pressure gradient >15mmHg during exercise
- Peak pulmonary arterial systolic pressure >60mmHg during exercise

Patients with positive results at stress echocardiography should be considered for balloon mitral valvuloplasty (or mitral valve surgery if unsuitable) even if resting echocardiography demonstrates only moderate MS.

Cardiovascular magnetic resonance

Cardiovascular magnetic resonance (CMR) can add significant information in selected valve patients, though is rarely a first line investigation for
assessment of valvular heart disease.

CMR is particularly useful for:
- Accurate and reproducible quantification of LV volume and function
- Accurate quantification of flow and regurgitant volume
- Precise anatomical information—direct planimetry of valve area,
  accurate outflow tract anatomy, localization of sub or supra-valvar
  stenosis (Fig. 2.21)
- Good views of difficult valves–especially the pulmonary valve
- The extent of any myocardial scar (e.g. infarction) and potential for
  improvement with revascularization.

Flow measurement

Through-plane flow

Flow through the image slice can be measured passing allowing quantification of both forward and regurgitant flow (Fig. 2.22), from which
regurgitant fraction can be calculated. Peak velocity can also be measured,
though temporal resolution is inferior to echocardiography. Planimetry of
stenotic valves is usually more accurate.

In-plane flow

Velocity can be measured within an image slice, allowing measurement
and visualization of velocities along the entire length of the flow jet. This is
particularly useful for stenotic lesions.

Limitations

- Some patients are unsuitable for cardiovascular magnetic resonance
  (CMR; pacemakers, cranial aneurysm clips etc). Prosthetic valves and
  stents are safe, though create a small localized artefact.
- Spatial resolution is lower than for echocardiography [particularly
  (TOE)] and fine detail of valve anatomy may be missed.
- Turbulent flow in very high velocity jets (>4m/s) can introduce errors
  in flow measurement.
- Temporal resolution of velocity measurements is lower than
  echocardiography (typically 25–40ms compared to 2–5ms) and CMR
  may underestimate the true peak velocity.
- Correct velocity settings are important for accurate flow
  measurement.

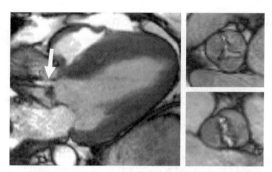

Fig. 2.21 CMR imaging in aortic stenosis. Left: a narrow high velocity jet (arrowed) in the LVOT (3-chamber) view. Top right: 'en-face' view through a stenotic trileaflet aortic valve—the area can be directly traced. Bottom right: 'en-face' view of a bicuspid stenotic aortic valve. From *Oxford Handbook of Cardiovascular Magentic Resonance* (2010) edited by Myerson, Francis and Neubauer.

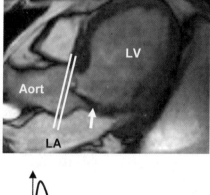

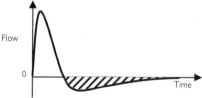

Fig. 2.22 Top: LVOT view showing aortic regurgitant jet (arrowed) and position of the image slice for flow measurement (parallel lines). Bottom: resulting flow graph over one cardiac cycle, showing moderate AR. The hatched area represents the volume of regurgitation.

Cardiac catheterization

The requirement for cardiac catheterization depends upon the patient profile, likely need for intervention and accuracy of non-invasive data.

Cardiac catheterization can include assessment of:
- Coronary arteries—usually as a preoperative assessment or to investigate LV dysfunction
- LV function—not routinely performed unless echocardiography limited
- Severity of MR and AR if non-invasive findings remain uncertain
- Aortic valve peak to peak gradient if non-invasive findings remain uncertain (see cautions below)
- Invasive measurement of pulmonary pressure, end-diastolic pressure and systemic venous pressure are possible
- Aortography allows assessment of aortic root anatomy and dimensions
- Fluoroscopy can be used to assess the degree of annular calcification.

Indications for cardiac catheterization

Suspected ischaemic mitral regurgitation
Ischaemic MR secondary to remodelling of the LV may be fixed or dynamic. Revascularization rather than mitral valve surgery may be the most effective strategy.

To exclude coronary artery disease prior to intervention:
- Males >40 years and post-menopausal women
- History of coronary artery disease
- Abnormal non-invasive investigation e.g. dobutamine stress echocardiography
- Chest pain suggestive of angina
- LV dysfunction
- Major cardiovascular risk factors.

Prosthetic valve dysfunction
Fluoroscopy can be invaluable in the assessment of prosthetic (metallic) valve dysfunction, where movement of the prosthetic leaflets can be assessed. In practice, echocardiography (particularly TOE) can provide useful information and fluoroscopy is reserved for when this is insufficient.

Cautions
The aortic valve should not be crossed in patients with severe AS since there is a significant risk of stroke as a result of embolism of calcified valve fragments.

Risk factors for cardiac disease

Ischaemic heart disease remains the most common cardiac disorder and should be actively identified or excluded in all patients with suspected valvular heart disease:
- Potential role in aetiology e.g. ischaemic MR
- Influence on intervention—additional revascularization increases surgical risk
- Influence on pathophysiology—more rapid deterioration possible
- Influence on medical therapy—may affect anticoagulation strategy.

Coronary angiography should be considered in all patients with the following characteristics, particularly if intervention is being considered:
- History of coronary artery disease—prior infarction/angina
- Symptoms typical for angina
- Abnormal exercise testing suggesting ischaemia
- LV systolic dysfunction
- Men >40 years of age
- Post-menopausal women
- More than one major cardiovascular risk factor.

Additional tests

Further information may be sought in selected patients:

Cardiac computed tomography

Multislice cardiac computed tomography (CT) can be used to exclude major coronary artery disease and may be useful for preoperative assessment in some patients. Examples include patients with significant valvular heart disease in whom there is a low risk of coronary artery disease, or where invasive coronary angiography would be hazardous (e.g. aortic valve IE with large vegetations and a root abscess).

Initial experience using cardiac CT to assess valve anatomy and function is limited and this mode of investigation is not currently recommended in routine practice.

Natriuretic peptides

Measurement of natriuretic peptides can be helpful in patients with heart failure, both as a diagnostic and prognostic tool, and for assessment of the effects of treatment. While the routine use of natriuretic peptides in valvular heart disease is not currently recommended, early evidence suggests they may have potential roles:
• Detection of the transition from compensated hypertrophy to dysfunction in AS with normal ejection fraction
• As a predictor of outcome in MR, especially in patients with minimal or no symptoms.

Radionuclide angiography

Serial assessment of ejection fraction is required in some patients with valvular heart disease and is a key factor in the timing of intervention. In the majority of patients, this assessment is performed using transthoracic echocardiography. If image quality is limited despite the use of contrast and CMR is unavailable, radionuclide angiography can provide an accurate and reproducible alternative.
• Sinus rhythm is necessary.
• Routine use in AR is not recommended.
• Myocardial perfusion imaging is insufficient to exclude coronary artery disease in patients with AS.
• Radionuclide angiography of the RV is more accurate than echocardiography in many cases.

Carotid artery disease

The combination of severe AS and significant carotid disease carries a particularly high operative risk.

Assessment of carotid anatomy is warranted in patients with a recent transient ischaemic attack or minor ischaemic stroke. Intervention may be required if significant stenosis of the internal carotid artery is detected—either as a staged procedure prior to elective valve surgery or as a combined intervention.

There are no clear guidelines for the preoperative management of the patient with a carotid bruit or abnormal Duplex ultrasound in the absence of symptoms. This finding will contribute to overall operative risk assessment but specific carotid intervention is generally best avoided. Vascular risk factor management remains appropriate.

General management

Introduction

The purpose of assessing a patient with valvular heart disease is to obtain information regarding the following:
- Diagnosis of valve lesion(s)
- Aetiology of valvular heart disease
- Quantification of severity
- Impact of valve lesion on cardiac function
- Need for medical therapy
- Need for surgical therapy
- Likely outcomes.

Once these factors have been clarified, the patient should be advised and educated on the appropriate management options, which may include:
- No further assessment or intervention required
- 'Watch and wait' with serial assessment
- Medical therapy and serial assessment
- Consideration of surgical intervention
- Immediate surgical intervention.

Clearly immediate surgical intervention is the priority in some patients with acute onset of severe valvular heart disease. However, the majority of patients are managed as out-patients and careful decision making regarding the timing of re-assessment and need for medical therapy is required.

Medical vs. surgical therapy

Medical therapy

Drug treatment for structural valvular heart disease is important but does not typically alter the progression of the lesion or delay definitive intervention. The main role is in the alleviation of symptoms and improvement of functional status. However, the presence of symptoms or signs of haemodynamic decompensation indicates that surgery may be necessary and medical therapy should not be used to alter this decision. Medical therapy may render the patient asymptomatic but long term outcome remains unpredictable.

Medical therapy directed at the underlying cause of secondary valvular heart disease (e.g. idiopathic dilated cardiomyopathy with functional MR) can reduce the severity and improve long term outcome if the underlying pathology is potentially reversible.

The main classes of drugs used in valvular heart disease are diuretics, vasodilators and rate limiting drugs, such as β-blockers. New drug therapies for valvular heart disease are limited e.g. statin and ACE inhibitor therapy for calcific AS.

A significant proportion of patients may be unsuitable for surgical intervention on the grounds of frailty, advanced age and co-morbidity. Medical therapy may be the only realistic option, although new trans-catheter techniques can play a role in selected cases. Medical therapy must be tailored to the individual patient and valve lesion: for example β-blockers can worsen AR by prolonging the diastolic period but are very helpful in MS as better rate control improves LV filling.

	Diuretics	Vasodilators	β-blockers
AS	With caution	With caution	Can relieve ischaemia
AR	Relieve congestion	Should be used	Contraindicated
MS	Relieve congestion	Not recommended	Should be used
Structural MR	With caution	Not recommended	Not recommended
Functional MR	Should be used	Should be used	Should be used
Ischaemic MR	Not recommended	Should be used	Should be used
TR	Should be used	Not recommended	Not recommended

Surgical therapy

The definitive treatment for the majority of symptomatic valvular heart disease is surgical repair or valve replacement. Careful patient selection and improved surgical technique and prosthesis design have led to excellent outcomes from valve surgery.

Balloon mitral valvuloplasty (see 📖 p.308) is an established initial alternative in patients with MS and newly available transcatheter techniques for AS and MR show promise.

The risks of the surgical procedure are difficult to quantify precisely but broadly relate to:
- Valve lesion
- Surgical complexity
- Need for additional bypass grafting
- LV and RV function
- Patient's physical status and preoperative mobility
- Comorbidity
- Surgical centre experience and outcomes.

Deciding when to refer a patient for surgery can be difficult. It is vital to ensure the patient has had sufficient explanation and education as to why an operation is required.

In many patients the early signs of decompensation, e.g. mild effort dyspnoea, allow adequate time to introduce the concept of surgical intervention. Further discussion can take place over several visits during surgical 'work-up'.

Surgery may need to be deferred for a short period if the patient has major imminent commitments given the impact of surgery on the patient's level of function in the postoperative period (average recovery time around three months). In many cases this will require careful assessment and planning to ensure no adverse effects of delay.

Aortic valve surgery

The overall in-hospital mortality for isolated aortic valve surgery is 3%, rising to 5% if concomitant bypass grafting is required. Most early in-hospital deaths relate to cardiac failure, stroke, haemorrhage and infection.

The long term survival is as follows:
- 75% at 5 years
- 60% at 10 years
- 40% at 15 years.

Patients receiving bioprosthetic valves have a higher mortality than those with a mechanical prosthesis but this reflects the increased age and co-morbidity of these patients.

Risk factors for increased mortality following aortic valve surgery include:
- Age (8-fold increase for a 75 year old compared to a 40 year old)
- Heart failure severity (New York Heart Association class)
- LV function
- Coronary artery disease
- Atrial fibrillation
- Re-do surgery
- Duration of surgery
- Female gender.

Mitral valve surgery

The overall in-hospital mortality of isolated mitral valve surgery is 4%, rising to 11% if concomitant bypass surgery is required. Early mortality is usually as a result of cardiac failure. As in aortic valve surgery, mortality associated with a bioprosthesis is generally higher, reflecting an older co-morbid patient group.

Long term survival is as follows:
- 82% at 1 year
- 68% at 5 years
- 55% at 10 years
- 35–50% at 15 years.

Risk factors for increased mortality following mitral valve surgery include:
- Age
- Aetiology—ischaemic MR has higher mortality
- Heart failure severity (New York Heart Association class)
- LV size and function
- Duration of surgery.

Complications of aortic valve surgery

- Bleeding.
- Tamponade.
- Myocardial infarction.
- Prolonged ventilation.
- Sternal infection.
- Renal dysfunction.
- Complete heart block: 2–3% require pacemaker.
- Stroke.
- Paraprosthetic regurgitation (rarely severe).
- IE—1% at 1 year and 3% at 5 years.
- Thromboembolism—dependent on valve type.
- Valve failure—dependent on valve type.

Complications of mitral valve surgery

As above, with the following exceptions:
- Pacemaker insertion is less likely
- Thromboembolism—more frequent than with aortic valves due to lower velocities across the valve
- Higher likelihood of atrial fibrillation.

Surgical risk assessment

The decision to proceed with surgery requires careful objective assessment of the patient's perioperative risk, integrated with local outcome data, the wishes of the patient, quality of life and overall life expectancy.

The European System for Cardiac Operative Risk Evaluation (EuroSCORE) is a validated assessment tool which estimates operative risk based on a number of readily available clinical variables:

- Age—increasing risk
- Gender—increased risk in females
- Chronic pulmonary disease—long term bronchodilator or steroid use
- Vascular disease—claudication, carotid stenosis >50%, aortic aneurysm (current or treated)
- Neurological disease—stroke limiting daily function
- Previous cardiac surgery
- Active IE
- Renal impairment—creatinine >200µmol/l
- Unstable angina—requiring intravenous nitrates
- Impaired LV—moderate or severe dysfunction
- Recent myocardial infarction—within 90 days
- Pulmonary hypertension—estimated pulmonary pressure >60mmHg
- Procedure other than isolated CABG
- Surgery on ascending aorta
- Post-infarction septal rupture
- Emergency case
- Critical perioperative condition: intra-aortic balloon pump, arrhythmia, ventilation, anuric renal failure.

A weighted score is given to any of these factors and the cumulative operative risk calculated. A more accurate model using the logistic co-efficient which may prevent underestimation from certain combinations of risk factors is also available.

For the full EuroSCORE risk calculator visit: http://www.euroscore.org/calc.html

Estimating risk in an individual patient is challenging and advice from an experienced surgeon invaluable. Many of the available risk calculators (EuroSCORE, Society of Thoracic Surgeons (STS) mortality risk score etc.) are based on registries of CABG and not valve intervention. Therefore, they are not universally applicable or accurate but provide an estimate which can be adjusted on an individual patient basis.

Disease monitoring

Most patients will require serial assessment of their symptoms, clinical status and disease severity, using a combination of clinical skills and echocardiography.

The timing of serial assessment is dependent on several factors, including:
• Valve lesion
• Severity—approaching threshold for intervention?
• Cardiac function—early signs of decompensation?
• Comorbidity—may affect tolerance of symptoms
• Rate of progression—evidence of rapid change in severity?
• Atypical symptoms—is the patient really asymptomatic?
• Support network—is primary care readily available?

An approximate guide to the timing of re-assessment in individual valve lesions is as follows:

Lesion	Mild	Moderate	Severe
AS	5 years	2 years	6 – 12 months
AR	2 years	1 year	6 months
MS	2 years	1 year	6 months
MR	2 years	1 year	6 months
TS	3 years	2 years	1 year
TR	3 – 5 years	2 – 3 years	1 – 2 years
PS	2 – 3 years	1 – 2 years	1 year
PR	2 – 3 years	1 – 2 years	1 year

At each visit the patient should be carefully assessed for changing symptoms or new evidence of decompensation.

Patient education

Patients with valvular heart disease should be advised on the following:
• Potential symptoms—and the need to report them early
• Prevention of IE – dental hygiene and skin care (see 🕮 p.388)
• Compliance with medical therapy – control of hypertension, warfarin
• Maintenance of good general health – impact of obesity or smoking
• Implications for non-cardiac surgery (see 🕮 p.320)
• Planning of pregnancy if appropriate (see 🕮 p.302 and p.332).

Role of guidelines

In contrast to most areas of cardiology, there is a very limited evidence base to guide the management of valvular heart disease, and a particular shortage of randomized double-blind multicentre controlled trials. Small scale studies of selected aspects of valvular heart disease have been undertaken: recent examples include the use of statin therapy in AS.

As a consequence, national and international bodies have developed guidelines to standardize the management of valvular heart disease.

American Heart Association/American College of Cardiology guidelines

The latest American guidelines were published in 2006 and can be accessed online at: ✒ http://circ.ahajournals.org

ACC/AHA 2006 Guidelines for the Management of Patients with Valvular Heart Disease: A Report of the American College of Cardiology/American Heart Association Task Force on Practice Guidelines (2006)

R. Bonow, B. A. Carabello, K. Chatterjee, A. C. de Leon, Jr, D. P. Faxon, M. D. Freed *et al. Circulation* 114:e84–e231.

This lengthy guideline (149 pages, 1066 references) covers all aspects of valvular heart disease with detailed sections on the management of valvular heart disease in pregnancy and congenital valvular heart disease in young adults.

European guidelines

The European Society of Cardiology published its updated guidelines in 2007 and these can be accessed online at:

ℜ http://www.escardio.org/knowledge/guidelines/Valvular-Heart-Disease.htm

Guidelines on the management of valvular heart disease: The Task Force on the Management of Valvular Heart Disease of the European Society of Cardiology (2007) A. Vahanian, H. Baumgartner, J. Bax, E. Butchart, R. Dion, G. Fillipatos, *et al. European Heart Journal*; 28:230–268.

This more streamlined document (39 pages, 232 references) contains guidance on the management of all common valvular heart disease as well as assessment and diagnosis, with additional sections on the management of valvular heart disease in pregnancy and during non-cardiac surgery.

The European Society of Cardiology has also published updated guidelines on the management of IE which can be accessed online at:

ℜ http://www.escardio.org/guidelines-surveys/esc-guidelines/Pages/infective-endocarditis.aspx

Guidelines on the prevention, diagnosis, and treatment of infective endocarditis (new version 2009) G. Habib, B. Hoen, P. Tornos, F. Thuny, B. Prendergast, I. Vilacosta *et al. European Heart Journal* 30:2369–2413.

Aortic stenosis

Introduction

AS is the third most common cardiovascular disease after hypertension and coronary artery disease and its incidence is increasing: it is the most common cause for aortic valve replacement and accounts for around 40,000 valve operations in Europe each year.

Patients often have a long asymptomatic period but deteriorate rapidly following the onset of symptoms. Timely diagnosis and intervention are therefore important to prevent progressive heart failure and death.

Epidemiology

AS is the most common valve lesion in developed nations, accounting for 43% of all valvular heart disease. The incidence is increasing with around 2% of adults >65 years of age having clinically significant valve obstruction, and by 85 years of age >5% have critical AS.

Women with severe AS present at an older age compared with men who have more co-morbidity and coronary artery disease.

Aetiology

AS is either congenital or acquired.

Causes include:
• Calcific degeneration (80%)
• Rheumatic heart disease (11%)
• IE
• Congenital lesions
• Paget's bone disease
• Ochronosis
• End stage renal failure
• Chronic inflammatory diseases
• Alkaptonuria.

Aetiology varies with age—stenosis of a bicuspid valve is more likely in a younger patient. Degenerative calcific AS will become even more common as rheumatic heart disease declines.

Degenerative AS

Calcific degeneration of the aortic valve is progressive with pathological findings similar to atherosclerosis. Slow accumulation of subendothelial lipoprotein accompanied by cellular infiltration and matrix deposition lead to leaflet thickening. Calcification progresses from the base of the cusps to the leaflet tips and reduces leaflet flexibility. Active bone formation may be seen in severe AS, particularly in patients with end stage renal failure.

Risk factors for AS mimic those of atherosclerosis: hypertension, diabetes, hyperlipidaemia, and smoking. Other emerging factors include the metabolic syndrome, inflammation (elevated high sensitivity C-reactive protein), and a possible genetic component.

Rheumatic AS

Inflammation of the valve leaflets following systemic infection with β-haemolytic streptococcus can lead to commissural fusion, calcification, and progressive stenosis. Although incidence is declining in developed nations, rheumatic heart disease still causes an estimated 250,000 deaths per year worldwide.

Congenital AS

Valve obstruction diagnosed in infancy or childhood is usually due to partial or complete absence of one or more commissures. Rarer causes include a subaortic membrane, muscular subaortic stenosis or supraval-vular stenosis and may be associated with genetic defects (e.g. Turner's syndrome, monosomy X) or other cardiac malformations (e.g. perimem-branous ventricular septal defect).

Bicuspid aortic valve

A bicuspid aortic valve (see 📖 p.12) is found in 2–3% of the population with 4:1 male preponderance. Most patients remain asymptomatic until ste-nosis develops later in adult life. Twenty percent of patients with a bicuspid aortic valve have an additional cardiovascular abnormality (e.g. aortic coarctation or patent ductus arteriosus).

Increased shear stress and mechanical wear and tear of a bicuspid valve lead to premature thickening and calcification identical to degeneration of a trileaflet valve. This so called sclerosis typically starts in the second decade of life with calcification from the fourth decade, the valve gradient increasing by 18mmHg per decade. As a consequence, patients with a bicuspid aortic valve typically present with valve stenosis five years before those with a trileaflet valve. Associated aortic root dilation is not uncommon and related to coexisting abnormalities of the elastic lamina: these patients have a 5-fold increase in the risk of aortic dissection (even after valve replacement).

Symptoms

The classical triad of symptoms is:
- Dyspnoea
- Angina
- Syncope on exertion.

Angina develops in up to two thirds of patients with significant AS, though only half of these have significant coronary artery disease.

Exercise-induced peripheral vasodilation causes syncope since the ventricle cannot increase cardiac output to maintain cerebral perfusion. Syncope may also be secondary to ventricular arrhythmias (provoked by ischaemia and myocardial fibrosis), or complete heart block due to calcification of adjacent conducting tissue.

Clinical signs

Findings depend on the severity of the stenosis and the ventricular response to outflow obstruction. Coexistent pathology (e.g. hypertension, vascular atherosclerosis) makes accurate assessment of severity challenging.

The hallmark of AS is a harsh crescendo–decrescendo systolic murmur, loudest in expiration, audible at the base and radiating to both carotids. Particularly high-pitched murmurs of AS may radiate to the apex and be mistaken for MR—the Gallavardin phenomenon. As stenosis progresses, the murmur peaks later in systole and the aortic component of the second heart sound is diminished or absent. Reduction in valve area of at least 50% is required to generate an audible murmur.

Clinical signs in aortic stenosis

Other clinical signs include:
- Slow rising low amplitude pulse—best felt at the carotid
- Reduced pulse pressure—<10% of patients
- Sustained apical impulse—due to LV hypertrophy
- Precordial thrill—unrelated to severity of stenosis
- Fourth heart sound - reflecting vigorous atrial systole
- Third heart sound—in LV systolic dysfunction
- Systolic click—in patients with a bicuspid valve.

Hypertension and aortic stenosis

Hypertension increases afterload as does aortic stenosis. Therefore patients with both are subject to a higher total LV load and may develop LV dysfunction and symptoms at an earlier stage.

There are additional implications for assessment in that hypertension will lead to reduced stroke volume (and hence transvalvular pressure drop) leading to underestimation of the severity of AS.

It is therefore important that the blood pressure is measured at the time of both clinical and echocardiographic assessment. If there is discordance between the apparent severity of AS and symptoms, then re-assessment after effective treatment of hypertension is appropriate.

Complications

The principal complication of AS is LV failure (Fig. 4.1).

Others include:
- IE—in up to 10% of patients
- Atrial fibrillation—can cause sudden increase in symptoms
- Ventricular arrhythmia—secondary to ischaemia and fibrosis
- Complete heart block—calcification of conduction tissue
- Bleeding tendency—epistaxis and ecchymoses in 20%
- Heyde's syndrome—GI bleeding due to angiodysplasia of the colon
- Embolic events—can occur rarely with heavily calcified valves
- Haemolytic anaemia—rare.

Natural history

Most patients remain asymptomatic for many years—morbidity and mortality are low and sudden death is rare (<1% per annum). Echocardiographic surveillance suggests an average reduction in valve area of 0.1cm^2 per year (0.3m/s increase in trans-aortic velocity, 7mmHg gradient) with a mean time from diagnosis to surgery >10 years. However, there is wide inter-individual variation.

Prognosis changes abruptly with the onset of symptoms (median survival: angina 45 months, exertional syncope 27 months, heart failure 11 months). Such symptoms are easily masked in the elderly.

Factors predictive of poor outcome include:
- Increasing age
- Risk factors for atherosclerosis
- Degree of valve calcification
- LV ejection fraction
- Annual increase in peak aortic velocity >0.45 m/s/yr
- Symptoms on formal exercise testing.

Asymptomatic very severe aortic stenosis

Asymptomatic patients with very severe aortic stenosis (peak aortic velocity >5.0m/s) have a poor prognosis with an increased risk of heart failure. Peak aortic velocity has been shown to correlate with survival, and patients with very high peak velocities, particularly if >5.5m/s, should be considered for early elective valve replacement even before symptoms develop.

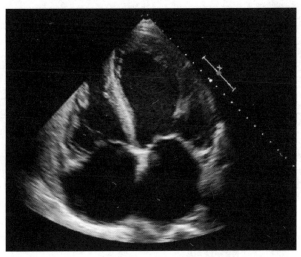

Fig. 4.1 End stage left ventricular dilation in severe aortic stenosis with an ejection fraction of 15%.

Exercise testing

Supervised exercise testing is safe in asymptomatic patients with AS. Patients may report no symptoms during routine daily activities but formal stress testing may identify unexpected limitation of exercise capacity or effort induced symptoms, such as dyspnoea or angina. As many as 50% of patients identified in this way will report symptoms within the next 12 months.

Assessment may be limited by co-morbidity or physical deconditioning—symptoms during exercise testing are more significant in a physically active patient <70 years of age; however it is reasonable to undertake exercise testing in older patients when intervention is being considered.

Exercise testing in a patient with significant AS is an unreliable tool for the assessment of coexistent coronary artery disease since angina, ST segment depression and hypotension can all occur in patients with severe AS and normal coronary arteries.

Criteria for a positive exercise test in asymptomatic AS (Bruce protocol):
- Limiting dyspnoea, chest discomfort or dizziness
- ST depression >5mm
- Non-sustained or sustained ventricular tachycardia
- Fall in systolic blood pressure >20mmHg from baseline.

The test should only be undertaken under appropriate medical supervision with close monitoring of ECG and blood pressure.

Initial investigations

In an asymptomatic patient, AS may be suspected on the basis of incidental clinical findings such as a murmur. Confirmation of the diagnosis requires echocardiography but investigations such as an ECG and chest X-ray are important to exclude other co-morbidity.

ECG in AS

The ECG may be entirely normal in mild AS. Progressive LV hypertrophy (Fig. 4.2) in moderate and severe AS manifests with:

• Large dominant R waves in I, aVL, V3-6
• Lateral ST segment and T wave abnormalities
• Left bundle branch block
• Left axis deviation.

Additional conduction tissue disease (first, second or third degree AV block) may also be seen.

Chest X-ray in AS

The heart size is normal. Calcification of the aortic annulus may be observed on an over-penetrated film. Post-stenotic dilation of the aorta (more common with bicuspid aortic valve) may be noted (Fig. 4.3), and coarctation (aortic contour abnormality and rib notching) should be excluded.

Differential diagnosis

Hypertension may be associated with angina, LV hypertrophy and a systolic murmur but without the other clinical signs typical of AS. Benign murmurs with an associated carotid bruit can also cause confusion.

Hypertrophic cardiomyopathy, PS and supravalvular aortic stenosis may produce similar ejection systolic murmurs—although skilled clinical examination can distinguish between these, echocardiographic assessment is usually required.

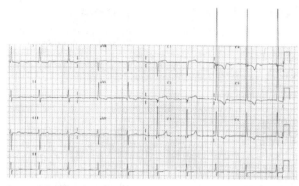

Fig. 4.2 ECG in severe AS—marked LV hypertrophy with repolarization abnormalities and prolonged PR interval.

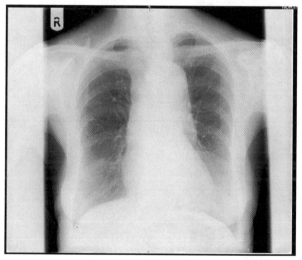

Fig. 4.3 Chest X-ray showing a dilated aortic root.

Echocardiographic assessment

The accuracy and reliability of two-dimensional and Doppler echocardiography in the assessment of AS has obviated the need for invasive haemodynamic measurement in most patients. Echocardiography is the investigation of choice to assess the aetiology, severity, LV diastolic and systolic performance, and associated cardiac abnormalities.

Valve morphology

Transthoracic two-dimensional echocardiography can assess the number, orientation, mobility, and calcification of the aortic valve leaflets in most patients. Transoesophageal imaging gives excellent views in almost all patients (Fig. 4.4).

The shape, symmetry, and motion of the valve leaflets is first assessed in the parasternal long axis position: this is also the ideal position to measure the diameter of the LV outflow tract. The parasternal short axis window affords good views of the aortic valve. In patients with limited parasternal windows, a similar short axis view can be achieved from the subcostal position. In many cases it is possible to directly planimeter the valve area from a single systolic frame although care must be taken to visualize the leaflet tips to ensure the true orifice is measured.

Grading of calcification

The following scoring system for the degree of calcification has been proposed (Fig. 4.5):
1. No calcification
2. Mild calcification—isolated small spots
3. Moderate calcification—multiple larger spots
4. Severe calcification—extensive thickening/calcification of all cusps

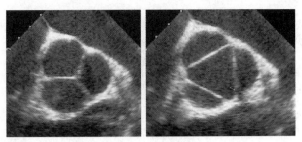

Fig. 4.4 Normal trileaflet aortic valve on transoesophageal echocardiography.

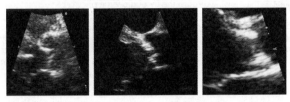

Fig. 4.5 Examples of mild, moderate and severe calcification of the aortic valve.

Doppler assessment

The accuracy of mean and instantaneous peak pressure gradients across a stenotic aortic valve derived using Doppler assessment (Fig. 4.6) has been well validated against direct invasive measurements. Typically, a catheter-derived pressure gradient is lower than that obtained with Doppler echocardiography due to the phenomenon of pressure recovery in the aorta. Cardiac output and stroke volume are also important determinants of the measured gradient.

The modified Bernoulli equation can be used to convert the peak velocity measured to a peak pressure drop:

Pressure drop = 4 × peak velocity²

Estimating valve area

Using the principle of conservation of energy, it is practical to estimate the valve area by assuming the volume of blood crossing the aortic valve is the same as that flowing through the LV outflow tract.

The valve area is calculated using the continuity equation (see 📖 p.62). Careful measurement of flow (Fig. 4.7) and outflow tract diameter are vital. Importantly, serial assessment should take into account the previously used LVOT area, as this rarely changes with time. Any Doppler measurement is sensitive to the angle of alignment with flow and care must be taken to ensure alignment within 15° of the jet.

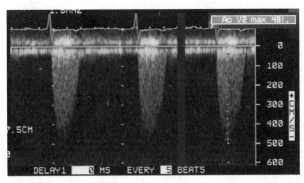

Fig. 4.6 Continuous wave Doppler in severe aortic stenosis—peak velocity nearly 5m/s. See also **Plate 6**.

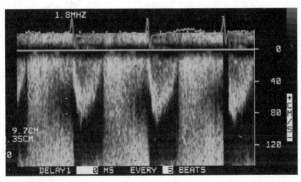

Fig. 4.7 Pulsed wave Doppler in LV outflow tract confirming normal velocity below the aortic valve.

LV size and function

LV cavity dimensions in systole and diastole along with septal and posterior wall thickness are measured from the parasternal long axis view via either M-mode assessment or direct measurement from a two-dimensional echocardiography still frame.

Systolic function of the LV is assessed using two-dimensional visual assessment and calculation of the ejection fraction with Simpson's bi-plane method if adequate endocardial border definition is achieved. Wall motion abnormalities should also be noted. Three-dimensional assessment of LV volumes and ejection fraction can also be utilized.

Impairment of LV diastolic function and elevated LV end diastolic pressure are important in the pathophysiology of AS and these should be assessed with available methodologies.

Associated abnormalities

A full echocardiographic dataset will also include assessment of:
- Structure and function of the remaining cardiac valves
- Estimation of peak RV systolic pressure
- Quantification of RV function
- Aortic root, ascending aorta and sinotubular junction
- Possible associated coarctation of the aorta
- Diameter of the descending abdominal aorta and presence of atheroma.

Transthoracic vs. transoesophageal echocardiography

It is feasible to derive accurate Doppler measurements and two-dimensional assessment of the aortic valve using transthoracic echocardiography in the majority of patients.

For those with limited transthoracic windows, or where there is doubt over the morphology of the aortic valve, then transoesophageal imaging affords excellent views in virtually all patients. Planimetry of the valve orifice is more accurate although care must be taken to ensure the image recorded is of the leaflet tips to avoid overestimation (Fig. 4.8).

Transoesophogeal Doppler assessment of the aortic valve is more difficult, requiring a deep transgastric position for appropriate alignment of the imaging plane which may be uncomfortable for patients (even when sedated).

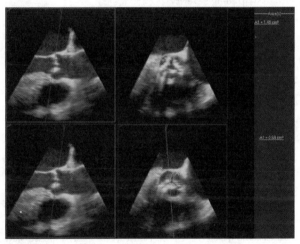

Fig. 4.8 Planimetry of the aortic valve is only accurate if the leaflet tips are in view—in the top panels the short axis cut is too low and the area overestimated compared to the true area shown in the lower panels.

Grading severity

Severity of AS is categorized according to the transaortic peak velocity, the mean and peak pressure gradient and the calculated valve area. Additional assessment using planimetry may also be useful.

A combination of these indices (combined with clinical assessment) determines final classification.

Criteria	Mild	Moderate	Severe
Peak instantaneous velocity (m/s)	< 3.0	3.0 – 4.0	> 4.0
Peak pressure drop (mmHg)	< 35	35 – 65	> 65
Mean pressure drop (mmHg)	<25	25 – 40	> 40
Valve area (cm^2)	2.0 – 1.5	1.5 – 1.0	< 1.0

Pitfalls in grading severity

Additional pathology may complicate echocardiographic assessment.

Overestimation of severity:
• Transaortic flow and velocity are increased in moderate or severe AR
• Peak velocity may also be increased in patients with high cardiac output or a small aortic root.

Underestimation of severity:
• LV systolic dysfunction: peak aortic velocity is dependent on LV contraction
• Poor alignment of the Doppler beam (Fig. 4.9).

The continuity equation to assess aortic valve area enables accurate assessment in these situations.

Beat-to-beat variation in peak Doppler signals is inevitable in the patient with atrial fibrillation. The highest obtainable velocities are used or an average over 5 to 10 cardiac cycles.

It is also critical to ensure that the gradient measured is that through the aortic valve—separating the signal from other systolic flow requires care—particularly with eccentric MR flowing under the anterior leaflet and close to the aortic sampling point.

A subaortic membrane can be hard to detect—serial pulsed wave sampling along the LV outflow tract should identify acceleration.

Low gradient severe AS with normal ejection fraction

Some patients (typically elderly females with long standing hypertension) present with symptomatic AS and a transvalvar gradient of only 30–40mmHg but a valve area <1.0cm². Such patients are likely to have severe AS with a small stroke volume as a result of cardiac hypertrophy and a small LV cavity.

Additional imaging

If the findings of transthoracic echocardiography are inconsistent with the clinical findings or there is persistent doubt regarding the severity of AS, then transoesophageal imaging will allow more accurate assessment of LV outflow tract diameter and valve morphology.

Alternative options include cardiac computed tomography (which also provides useful information on the degree of calcification), CMR imaging and three dimensional echocardiography (Fig. 4.10).

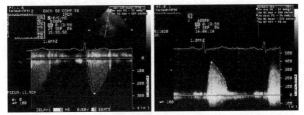

Fig. 4.9 The importance of accurate Doppler assessment. In the left hand panel the peak velocity measured from the apex is 2.8m/s. When re-assessed in the right parasternal position (flow is now towards the transducer), the peak velocity is in fact 4m/s—significantly altering the grading of severity.

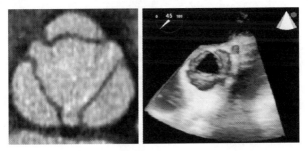

Fig. 4.10 Aortic valve imaging with cardiac CT and real-time 3D TOE.

Invasive assessment

Cardiac catheterization is rarely necessary for the diagnosis of AS given the accuracy and ubiquity of echocardiography. Only in exceptional cases (where echocardiographic data are insufficient or coexistent mitral valve disease complicates assessment) are direct measurement of LV pressure and aortic valve gradient required.

It is also important to appreciate differences in the measurements obtained with both techniques. Direct pressure measurement during pull-back of a catheter through the aortic valve assesses the difference in peak LV and peak aortic pressure (the peak-to-peak gradient), whereas continuous wave Doppler assesses the difference in peak instantaneous velocity (or peak pressure drop) (Fig. 4.11). The peak-to-peak gradient is always lower—a valve with a peak velocity of 4m/s across it will have a peak-to-peak gradient of around 40mmHg but an echocardiographic peak pressure drop of 60mmHg.

Trauma to the diseased valve during attempts to cross it carries a risk of systemic embolism of valve fragments—up to 20% of patients will have new ischaemic lesions on cerebral MRI, with 3–4% sustaining a stroke. The safest approach is with a Judkins right or Amplatzer left coronary catheter and a soft tipped 0.035inch straight guidewire (Fig. 4.12). Alternative approaches, including trans-septal puncture via the right atrium or direct apical puncture, are rarely used.

Current European and American guidelines recommend that retrograde catheterization of the LV through a stenotic aortic valve should be undertaken with caution and only in situations where echocardiographic assessment is inconclusive.

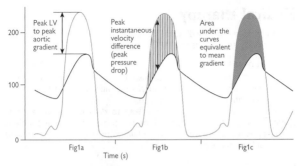

Fig. 4.11 Explanation of differences in catheter- and Doppler-derived measurements in aortic stenosis.

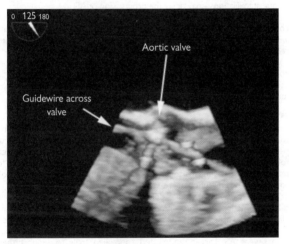

Fig. 4.12 Crossing a stenotic aortic valve with an Amplatzer left coronary catheter and a straight 0.035" guidewire.

Medical therapy

There are no specific medical therapies which prevent the development of AS or delay its progression.

General measures

Many patients with AS have coexistent coronary artery disease—preventative measures (aspirin, statins, ACE inhibitors, and β blockers) apply, along with general lifestyle advice.

The onset of atrial fibrillation can lead to dramatic deterioration in symptoms as the additional cardiac output provided by atrial systole is lost. Aggressive approaches to maintain sinus rhythm (e.g. vigorous control of hypertension) are appropriate.

Statin therapy in AS

The pathophysiology of AS and atherosclerosis is similar and it seems intuitive that the effects of statins—inhibition of inflammation, antioxidant, plaque stabilisation—may delay the progression of AS.

However, despite promising preclinical data, large randomized controlled studies have shown no benefit of high dose statins in patients with at least moderate AS. Much earlier treatment may be required to reduce inflammation and lipid deposition to influence outcome.

In practice, many patients with AS have coexistent hypertension, coronary artery disease, diabetes or hyperlipidaemia and warrant statin therapy. Current guidelines do not advocate routine use of statin therapy for AS alone.

ACE inhibitors

Traditional teaching is that angiotensin-converting enzyme (ACE) inhibitors are contra-indicated in AS due to the risks of syncope as a result of peripheral vasodilation. In reality, many patients (even those with severe AS) tolerate ACE inhibition safely. Given the effect of AS on the LV, measures to preserve normal ventricular function and prevent or delay progression to frank systolic dysfunction are attractive.

A number of animal studies demonstrate that ACE inhibitors improve diastolic function and maintain normal systolic function in AS. Small scale clinical studies also support the use of ACE inhibitors to treat hypertension in patients with moderate AS and improve functional capacity in those with severe AS. Larger randomized controlled trials to support their routine use are awaited.

Surveillance

Once the diagnosis of AS is established, appropriate follow up with access to surveillance echocardiography should be arranged.

General measures

Patients should be made aware of the potential symptoms of AS and encouraged to report these as early as possible.

Patients should remain active and are safe to exercise if this does not provoke symptoms. Patients with mild AS can participate in all competitive sports but require annual surveillance. Those with moderate stenosis should refrain from competitive sports involving high dynamic or static muscular demands, such as body-building, boxing, skiing, cycling and running. Supervised exercise stress testing may be required to document safe effort capacity.

Patients with severe AS should not undertake rigorous exercise.

There are no specific restrictions to driving unless AS is complicated by angina, syncope or heart failure, where restrictions do apply.

Asymptomatic AS should not restrict travel by air but professional aviation bodies are only likely to grant licences to patients with mild stenosis.

Serial review

Annual assessment of the asymptomatic patient following initial diagnosis is recommended to document the degree and rate of change of AS before deciding on review frequency.

Follow up arrangements thereafter depend on individual patient characteristics (e.g. age, degree of calcification, co-morbidity, level of activity). As an approximate guide, the following intervals are recommended for clinical and echocardiographic review.

Severity	Minimum review frequency
Mild AS	5 years
Moderate AS	2 years
Severe AS	6 – 12 months

More frequent review is appropriate in the presence of symptoms or progressive clinical or echocardiographic findings.

Indications for surgery

The optimal treatment is relief of outflow obstruction by means of aortic valve replacement. Virtually all patients with symptomatic severe AS should be considered for surgery.

Clear surgical indications include:
• Symptomatic severe AS
• Asymptomatic patients with severe AS and exercise induced symptoms or hypotension
• Asymptomatic patients with moderate or severe AS undergoing CABG, aortic root surgery, or replacement of another valve.

Although operative mortality of aortic valve replacement is low, the long term morbidity and mortality associated with a prosthetic valve are not small. Major complications are seen in 2–3% of patients per year and death related to prosthetic valve complications occurs in 1% per year. Careful consideration of the risk–benefit ratio of surgical intervention is mandatory, especially in asymptomatic patients.

Additional indications for surgery in asymptomatic patients include:
• Asymptomatic patients with severe AS and LV ejection fraction <50% without alternative aetiology
• Asymptomatic patients with severe AS, moderate to severe calcification and a change in peak velocity >0.3m/s per year
• Asymptomatic patients with very severe AS – peak velocity >5m/s (see 📖 p.103).

Surgery may also be considered in patients with severe AS associated with:
• Ventricular arrhythmias on exercise testing
• Excess LV hypertrophy (>15mm wall thickness) with no alternative cause (e.g. hypertension).

Aortic stenosis with left ventricular impairment

AS and LV systolic impairment frequently coexist. Underlying aetiology is often uncertain and may be a combination of the long-term effects of outflow obstruction and concomitant coronary artery disease with or without myocardial infarction. Moderate AS with associated LV impairment may be difficult to distinguish from severe AS with fixed obstruction and is often termed 'pseudo-severe AS'.

Echocardiographic assessment is difficult since measures of trans-aortic flow velocity and peak pressure drop are dependent on LV function. These measures are reduced in the presence of LV impairment resulting in underestimation of the severity of stenosis. Determination of valve area using the flow-independent continuity equation remains valid.

Low gradient, low flow aortic stenosis

This is defined as:
- LV ejection fraction <40%
- Mean pressure drop <30mmHg
- Effective orifice area <1.0cm^2.

It is therefore vital that all echocardiographic assessment of AS includes a calculation of valve area to allow identification of patients with low gradient, low flow AS.

Diagnosis and assessment

The key question is whether the AS is genuinely severe and the LV dysfunction secondary, or the AS is only moderate and the LV impaired due to infarction or an alternative cause. The likelihood of recovery of the ventricle is higher if the cause is AS, although in some cases myocardial fibrosis is severe and little ventricular recovery possible.

The use of low dose dobutamine, a selective β1-adrenoceptor agonist, identifies LV contractile reserve and can aid grading of the severity of AS. An infusion of 5μg/kg/min is slowly increased up to a maximum of 20μg/kg/min with careful monitoring.

If the stenosis is truly severe then the rise in mean pressure drop is accompanied by only a small rise in effective orifice area: the ventricular performance has improved generating a higher pressure drop through a relatively fixed stenotic orifice.

In moderate AS, the rise in mean pressure drop is less marked with a larger rise in effective orifice area: ventricular performance has improved and greater trans-valvular flow leads to increased opening of the valve, so there is no major rise in pressure drop across the valve.

In practical terms, an increase in the mean pressure drop to above 30mmHg at any point is suggestive of severe AS.

More important than the change in pressure drop is the change in performance of the LV. If the ejection fraction improves and the velocity–time integral of trans-aortic flow on continuous wave Doppler (stroke volume) increases by 20% or more, then the surgical risk and long-term outcome is considerably better—5% operative mortality compared to 32% in those where LV function does not improve.

Indications for surgery in low gradient, low flow AS:
During dobutamine infusion:
• Severe AS—mean pressure drop >30mmHg and area <1.2cm^2
• Increase in stroke volume >20%.

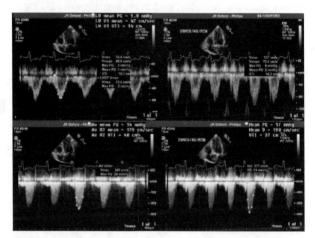

Fig. 4.13 Example of pseudo-severe aortic stenosis. In the left hand panel the Doppler data suggests severe aortic stenosis but after dobutamine infusion the stroke volume has increased without a marked increase in the peak velocity (right hand panel).

AS with MR

The detection of more than mild MR in patients requiring aortic valve surgery is common—around 60% have a degree of MR and in 15% this is severe.

Pathophysiology

AS with MR may be the consequence of rheumatic heart disease, degenerative disease of both valves, LV dysfunction due to AS leading to functional MR, or congenital AS with mitral valve prolapse.

Severe AS increases any pre-existing MR as the stroke volume will preferentially pass through the regurgitant valve rather than through the stenotic orifice. A further effect of this reduced forward stroke volume is to lead to a decrease in peak and mean trans-aortic pressure drop and potential under-estimation of the severity of AS. As in chronic isolated MR, the off-loading effect of regurgitant flow is to 'flatter' the LV leading to masking of early systolic dysfunction which may have already become apparent in isolated AS.

Additional consequences of MR include the development of atrial fibrillation—the loss of atrial systole leads to impaired filling of a hypertrophied ventricle further reducing stroke volume and trans-aortic velocity. In significant MR, further changes include pulmonary hypertension and TR—usually seen when LV failure supervenes.

Management

If there is no significant mitral valve pathology, annulus dilation or abnormal ventricular geometry then mitral valve intervention is not required. Functional MR often improves significantly once the LV outflow obstruction is relieved and ventricular pressure falls.

Double valve replacement markedly increases perioperative risk over isolated aortic valve replacement but should be considered in:

- Severe MR (effective regurgitant orifice $>30mm^2$)
- Minimal co-morbidities
- Otherwise low operative risk
- High potential for mitral valve repair.

AS in patients needing CABG

Patients with severe AS requiring CABG should undergo simultaneous valve replacement since long-term mortality is lower than with CABG alone. Conversely, patients with mild AS should not undergo valve replacement at the time of CABG since combined surgery carries higher risk.

The majority of patients with moderate AS who require CABG benefit from combined surgery, although the rate of progression of AS, co-morbidity and projected risk of repeat surgery should be considered for each individual patient. Initial CABG with future transcatheter aortic valve implantation may become a useful treatment strategy in this group.

Isolated valve replacement may relieve symptoms and prolong life in the patient with severe symptomatic AS and associated inoperable coronary artery disease, albeit at high operative risk. A hybrid approach combining surgical valve replacement and percutaneous revascularization may be appropriate in selected patients.

Management algorithm for severe aortic stenosis

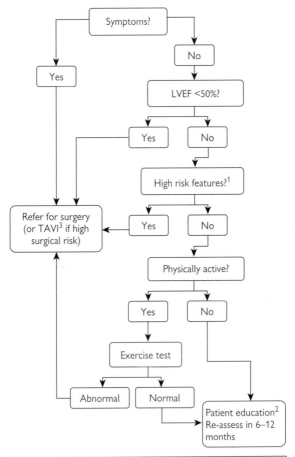

1 Severe valve calcification, peak jet velocity increase >0.3m/s in 1 year
2 Advise on symptoms and need for early reporting
3 Transcatheter aortic valve implantation

Aortic regurgitation

Introduction

AR may result from pathology affecting the valve leaflets or as a secondary consequence of disease of the aortic root. Chronic regurgitation is often well tolerated but acute regurgitation usually requires early intervention. As in other valvular heart disease, prevalence increases with age.

Epidemiology

AR is considerably less frequent than AS. Recent data suggest a prevalence of at least mild AR in 19% of men and 20% of women. There is a clear relation to age; 4% of men <30 years of age have AR compared with 39% of men aged >80 years (Fig. 5.1).

Aetiology

AR may be a primary lesion of the valve leaflets or secondary to disruption of the aortic root.

Primary valve lesion
- Rheumatic valvular heart disease
- IE
- Degenerative valvular heart disease
- Traumatic leaflet rupture (usually secondary to deceleration injury)
- Congenital abnormalities
  - Bicuspid aortic valve
  - Sub-arterial ventricular septal defect
  - Subaortic stenosis
- Iatrogenic
- Rheumatoid arthritis
- Systemic lupus erythematosus (Libman–Sacks endocarditis)

Aortic root pathology
- Aortic root dilation
  - Marfan's syndrome
  - Osteogenesis imperfecta
  - Syphilis
  - Ankylosing spondylitis
  - Reiter's syndrome
- Aortic dissection
- Hypertension

Primary valve abnormalities are falling in incidence and AR due to root pathology now accounts for >50% of cases.

IE and aortic dissection are the two most common causes of acute AR.

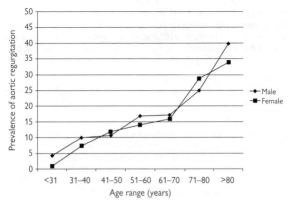

Fig. 5.1 Prevalence of unsuspected and significant aortic regurgitation. Data from Stefano G. (2008) *Journal of the American Society of Echocardiography* 21:38–42.

Rheumatic valvular heart disease

Leaflet fibrosis and cusp fusion lead to retraction from the zone of apposition with resultant valvular regurgitation. Rheumatic valvular heart disease remains the most common cause of AR in developing countries but is rare in Europe and the US.

Degenerative valvular heart disease

Calcific degeneration can lead to both AS and AR, but AR is seldom the dominant lesion.

Bicuspid aortic valve

The abnormal shear stress associated with flow through a bicuspid valve results in premature leaflet degeneration. While AS is the most frequent outcome, AR or mixed aortic valve disease may also result as a consequence of leaflet fibrosis, retraction or prolapse, particularly in younger patients. Associated abnormalities of the tunica media may cause additional aortic root dilation (Fig. 5.2).

Sub-arterial ventricular septal defect

Defects of the inter-ventricular septum can lead to prolapse of the aortic valve leaflets and resultant AR. This scenario typically accompanies a sub-arterial defect when there is reduced support for the right- or non-coronary cusp. Systolic flow through the ventricular septal defect drags the valve leaflet into the RV with sustained displacement and resultant AR (Fig. 5.3). AR progressively increases with age and the risk of IE is high.

Subaortic stenosis

Fixed stenosis below the aortic valve is usually due to a fibrous membrane or muscular narrowing of the LV outflow tract. A high velocity jet is directed at the aortic valve, with consequent trauma and leaflet scarring. More than 50% of patients with subaortic stenosis have AR, which is moderate or severe in 12%.

Aortic root dilation

The anatomy of the aortic root is complex - the aortic valve does not have a distinct circular annulus but a crown shaped area of connection between the valve leaflets and aortic wall (see 📖 p.6) Dilation of the aortic root leads to separation of the valve leaflets, failure of complete apposition and consequent AR.

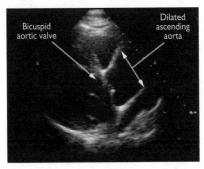

Fig. 5.2 Transthoracic echocardiogram demonstrating marked dilation of the ascending aorta in a patient with a bicuspid aortic valve.

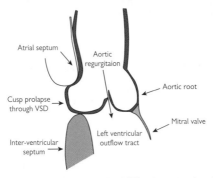

Fig. 5.3 Sub-arterial ventricular septal defect (VSD) with associated aortic regurgitation.

Aortic dissection

Acute dissection of the proximal aorta (type A) is associated with acute AR in 40–70% of patients. The mechanism of AR is variable: if the dissection arises within an already dilated aorta then AR may be secondary to root dilation itself. Alternatively, the dissection plane may disrupt leaflet attachment with resultant prolapse and AR. Finally, the dissection flap itself may prolapse through the aortic valve and prevent complete leaflet closure without damage to the leaflets themselves.

Iatrogenic

Iatrogenic AR may arise as result of trauma to the valve leaflets during passage of guidewires or catheters or following balloon valvuloplasty for AS. AR may also develop as a result of technical failure of aortic valve repair or replacement.

Symptoms

Chronic AR may remain asymptomatic for many years as the ventricle copes with increased stroke volume. Eventually, these compensatory mechanisms fail with development of symptoms:

- Dyspnoea—initially on effort, then at rest
- Awareness of cardiac activity
- Prominent or bounding heart beat
- Chest discomfort
- Angina.

Acute AR leads to acute dyspnoea due to pulmonary oedema—associated chest or back pain suggests the possibility of underlying aortic dissection.

Clinical signs

The increased stroke volume in AR leads to a large variety of clinical signs, many of which remain eponymous following their original description. The range of signs in an individual patient depends upon the regurgitant volume, degree of remodelling and performance of the LV.

Pulse and peripheral signs

As the severity of AR increases the diastolic blood pressure falls and pulse pressure widens (defined as a difference between the systolic and diastolic pressure >50mmHg or more than 50% of the systolic pressure).

Other clinical signs relate to the development of ventricular failure and may include:

- Pulmonary oedema
- Elevated venous pressure
- Peripheral oedema
- Low output state with hypotension
- Cardiogenic shock.

Murmur

Regurgitation of blood from the aorta to the LV results in a high-pitched blowing diastolic murmur which decreases in intensity through diastole.

The murmur may be easier to detect with the patient sitting forward and in end-expiration, listening in the left fourth intercostal space. Manoevures to increase arterial resistance (e.g. inflating sphygmomanometer cuffs on both arms above systolic pressure) will enhance the murmur. A systolic murmur (secondary to increased stroke volume or coexistent AS, perhaps with a bicuspid valve) or late-diastolic apical murmur (the Austin–Flint murmur, related to the impact of AR on the endocardium) may also be audible.

The timing and duration of the murmur (but not its intensity) correlate with the severity of AR. Patients with acute severe AR have a holo-diastolic murmur which is often quiet and difficult to detect.

Natural history

Outlook for patients with asymptomatic chronic AR is good: <6%/year progress to symptoms or signs of LV dysfunction. Those with aortic root dilation or a bicuspid aortic valve may progress more rapidly.

Patients with symptoms, LV dilation or dysfunction have significant mortality risk:

- NYHA Class II—6%/yr
- NYHA Class III/IV—25%/yr.

Valve replacement should therefore be considered once there is evidence of symptoms or LV decompensation.

Eponymous signs

The following eponymous signs have been described:

Sign	Explanation
Austin Flint murmur	Mid-diastolic murmur not due to mitral stenosis
Becker sign	Enhanced retinal artery pulsation
Bozzolo sign	Pulsatile nasal mucosa
Corrigan pulse	Collapsing peripheral pulse
De Musset sign	Pulsatile head nodding
Dennison sign	Pulsatile cervix
Drummond sign	Pulsatile air expulsion when mouth is closed
Duroziez sign	To-and-fro femoral sound under compression
Gerhard sign	Pulsatile spleen
Hill sign	Higher systolic pressure in legs than in arm
Landolfi sign	Pulsatile pupils
Lincoln sign	Exaggerated foot movement with legs crossed
Mayne sign	Drop in diastolic pressure >15mmHg on arm elevation
Mueller sign	Pulsatile uvula
Quincke sign	Visible pulsation in capillary nail bed
Rosenbach sign	Pulsatile liver
Sherman sign	Prominent dorsalis pedis pulse in patients over 75
Traube sign	Loud systolic and diastolic sound over femorals

Initial investigations

Although the ECG and chest X-ray may be helpful, definitive diagnosis is achieved with echocardiography.

ECG

There are no diagnostic changes and the ECG may be normal. LV hypertrophy with ST repolarization changes and left axis deviation may accompany severe AR.

Chest X-ray

LV enlargement and/or dilation of the aorta may be seen and pulmonary congestion or oedema once symptoms develop (Fig. 5.4).

Differential diagnosis

The bounding pulse and wide pulse pressure characteristic of AR may accompany other disease states although an associated diastolic murmur would not be expected:
- Thyrotoxicosis
- Fever
- Anaemia
- Pregnancy
- Patent ductus arteriosus
- Cirrhosis
- Paget's disease of bone
- Multiple arteriovenous fistula.

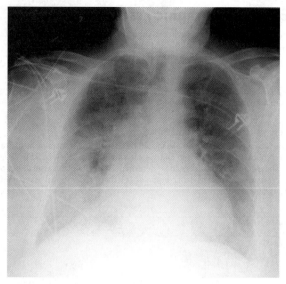

Fig. 5.4 Chest X-ray demonstrating severe bilateral pulmonary oedema and enlargement of the cardiac silhouette due to acute severe aortic regurgitation.

Echocardiographic assessment

Full echocardiographic assessment should include the following:
- Severity of AR—colour flow and Doppler
- Valve morphology and mechanism
- Aortic anatomy and dimensions
- LV diastolic and systolic dimensions
- LV ejection fraction
- Pulmonary arterial pressure
- Other valve lesions.

Left ventricular size and function

The size and shape of the LV should be assessed with careful measurement of cavity dimensions in end-systole and end-diastole (Fig. 5.5).

The ejection fraction should be determined using bi-plane assessment of end-diastolic and end-systolic volumes (or three-dimensional assessment if available: Fig 5.6).

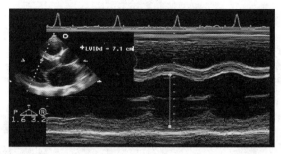

Fig. 5.5 The end-diastolic dimension of the LV. Care must be taken to ensure that the plane of measurement is perpendicular to the cavity and in end-diastole. In this case, the ventricle is severely dilated at 7.1cm (LVIDd = left ventricular internal dimension in diastole).

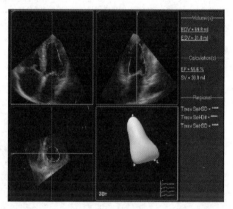

Fig. 5.6 Three-dimensional assessment of LV volume and ejection fraction. If accurate determination of ejection fraction is not possible using echocardiography then radionuclide ventriculography or cardiac magnetic resonance imaging provide a valid alternative. See also **Plate 7**.

Severity assessment—colour flow and Doppler

Colour flow Doppler is a highly sensitive method for the detection of AR which allows accurate visualization and quantification of the regurgitant jet (Fig. 5.7).

Vena contracta

The width of the narrowest portion of the regurgitant jet (which reflects the diameter of the regurgitant orifice) is known as the vena contracta; a width <0.3cm suggests mild AR and >0.6cm severe AR.

Jet width indexed to left ventricular outflow tract

A jet which occupies <25% of the width of the LV outflow tract suggests mild AR. Conversely, a wide jet occupying >65% indicates severe AR.

Pressure half time

The speed at which regurgitant velocity decays in diastole is proportional to the severity of AR—the pressure between the aorta and ventricle equalizes more rapidly in severe AR. The pressure half time is the time required for pressure across the valve to fall by 50% and is derived from measurement of the peak velocity and deceleration slope (Fig. 5.8).

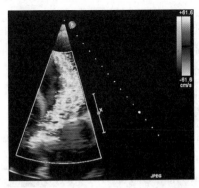

Fig. 5.7 Apical 5-chamber view demonstrating a wide jet of severe AR in the LV outflow tract extending to the apex. See also **Plate 8.**

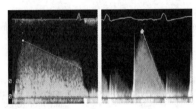

Fig. 5.8 The left hand panel shows mild AR with a shallow deceleration slope. The right hand panel shows severe AR with rapid deceleration (and increased density) of the signal.

Flow in the descending aorta

Significant AR results in retrograde aortic flow during diastole which may be detected in the ascending (suprasternal window) or descending aorta (suprasternal or subcostal window) using pulsed wave Doppler (Fig. 5.9).

Valve morphology

Transthoracic and transoesophageal echocardiography can identify the pathology underlying AR. A bicuspid valve, dilated aortic root, and IE with vegetations or cusp destruction can all be easily demonstrated (Fig. 5.10).

Aortic anatomy and dimensions

Careful measurement of aortic root dimensions is mandatory in any patient with AR (Fig. 5.11). A dilated aortic root may be the cause of AR and will have impact on subsequent surgical intervention.

Regurgitant volume and effective orifice area

Quantitative assessment of the regurgitant volume and effective orifice area can be undertaken using the PISA method (more commonly used in MR, see 📖 p.64). These measurements are more challenging in AR due to difficulties with consistent Doppler alignment and are consequently rarely used in routine assessment.

Associated abnormalities

Additional valvular heart disease, LV and RV function, and pulmonary arterial pressure should all be assessed in a patient with AR.

Transthoracic vs. transoesophageal echocardiography

Transoesophageal echocardiography (TOE) affords better views of the aortic valve and proximal aortic root aiding assessment of the severity and pathology of AR. Chronic AR can be safely monitored with serial transthoracic echocardiography but a TOE is often required if surgery is contemplated.

Emerging technology (e.g. real-time 3D TOE) can be of further assistance in difficult cases.

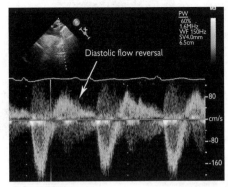

Fig. 5.9 Pulse wave Doppler (suprasternal window) of flow in the descending thoracic aorta. Flow reversal throughout the whole diastolic period (arrowed) indicates severe AR.

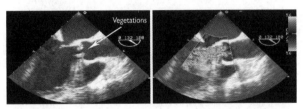

Fig. 5.10 Transoesophageal echocardiogram in aortic valve IE demonstrating large vegetations on both the non-coronary and right-coronary cusps. A diastolic image (left hand panel) shows a clear defect in the valve (arrowed) with resultant severe AR (right hand panel)—the colour flow signal occupies the entire LV outflow tract. See also **Plate 9**.

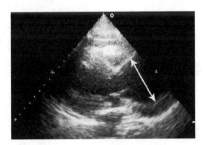

Fig. 5.11 Transthoracic frame in systole demonstrating a severely dilated aortic root.

Grading severity

The severity of AR is classified according to a combination of echocardiographic parameters:

	Mild	Moderate	Severe
Vena contracta	<0.3cm	0.3–0.6cm	>0.6cm
Jet width in LVOT	<25% LVOT	25–65% LVOT	>65% LVOT
Descending aorta flow	Brief early diastolic flow	←In-between→	Holodiastolic flow reversal
Pressure half time	>500ms	500–200ms	<200ms
Regurgitant volume	<30ml	30–60ml	>60ml
LV (chronic AR)	Normal size		Moderate or severe dilation with no other cause

Pitfalls in grading severity

- Eccentric jets entrain the walls of the LVOT or surface of the anterior mitral valve leaflet.
- Eccentric jets may prove difficult to align accurately for Doppler assessment.
- Assessment of the vena contracta and jet width depends upon the view chosen since the jet is not circular.
- Gain, colour scale, and Nyquist limits alter the colour flow pattern and affect assessment of severity: standard settings should be used to ensure consistency over serial studies.
- Remodelling of the LV may slow equalization of pressure across the valve—impact on the pressure half time may result in underestimation of the severity of chronic AR.

Exercise testing

There is no established role for exercise testing in determining the need for intervention in AR. However, since onset and progression of symptoms are usually gradual, patients may be sedentary and claim to be asymptomatic. Exercise testing may be useful to demonstrate symptoms and reduced effort tolerance, and provides a baseline for serial assessment.

Brain natriuretic peptide

Levels of BNP and NT-pro BNP correlate with the severity of AR and presence of symptoms. Rising levels may indicate progressive disease prompting repeat assessment (and possible need for intervention) but routine measurement of BNP does not feature in current guidelines.

Avoiding assessment error

Use all parameters to judge severity and avoid reliance on a single measurement.

AR jets are often eccentric—careful imaging using multiple views is required for full assessment.

Leaflet perforation and small vegetations may be difficult to visualize with transthoracic imaging—always consider transoesophageal assessment in IE.

Invasive assessment

Cardiac catheterization is seldom required for the diagnosis of AR, although coronary angiography is required in the majority of patients being considered for surgical treatment. At this assessment, aortography is often performed to further evaluate the AR and determine the diameter of the ascending and descending aorta. Left ventriculography and measurement of LV end-diastolic pressure can also be easily performed.

Medical therapy

Asymptomatic patients with mild or moderate AR do not require treatment unless there is coexistent hypertension. Asymptomatic patients with severe AR or progressive ventricular enlargement may benefit from vasodilator therapy (hydralazine, ACE inhibitors, or nifedipine) although supportive evidence is limited. Diuretics may palliate symptoms but should not be used to defer the need for intervention. β-blockers are relatively contra-indicated since prolongation of diastole will increase regurgitant volume.

Excessive reduction of diastolic blood pressure will reduce coronary blood flow in severe AR and careful titration of therapy is required.

General measures

Lifestyle measures to prevent hypertension and the development of coronary artery disease are appropriate (as in all valvular heart disease). Regular screening for hypertension is essential in AR with prompt treatment when detected.

Surveillance

General measures

Patients should be counselled and educated of the need to promptly report any changes in functional capacity.

Asymptomatic patients should remain active and can exercise if able to do so. Regular blood pressure checks are recommended.

The minimum frequency of clinical review is 12 months since early onset LV dysfunction (within 12–14 months) is often fully reversible once AR has been corrected.

Indications for surgery

Symptomatic patients should undergo surgery to repair or replace the aortic valve.

Surgery should also be considered in asymptomatic patients with:
• Progressive LV dysfunction—LV end diastolic diameter >7cm, LV end systolic diameter >5cm, LV ejection fraction <50%.
• Aortic root dilation >55mm (>50mm if bicuspid valve or >45mm in Marfan's syndrome).

Serial review

Severity	Minimum review frequency
Mild to moderate	12 months clinical review – echocardiography every 24 months
Severe	6 months if LVEDD > 60mm
Aortic root dilation	12 months if root > 40mm irrespective of severity

AR in patients needing CABG

Aortic valve surgery (repair if feasible) should be considered in any patient with at least moderate AR undergoing coronary artery bypass grafting; however, decisions should be made on an individual patient basis, according to the aetiology and duration of AR and the likelihood of progression.

Management algorithm for aortic regurgitation

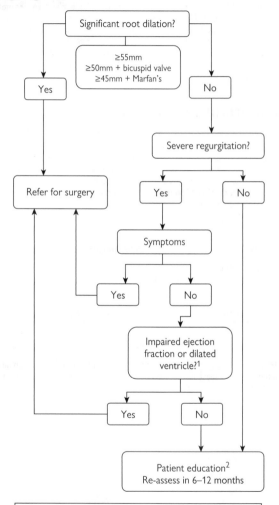

¹Ejection fraction ≤50%, left ventricular diastolic diameter >70mm
²advise on symptoms and need for early reporting

Mitral stenosis

Introduction

MS is now rare in Western societies due to the declining incidence of rheumatic fever. Worldwide, it remains an important cause of cardiovascular morbidity and mortality due to the higher prevalence of rheumatic valvular heart disease in developing countries and increased population migration.

Balloon mitral valvuloplasty has revolutionized management and remains an important interventional skill, particularly as patients may present abruptly (e.g. in pregnancy) and require swift relief of valve obstruction.

Epidemiology

MS is the least frequent valve lesion, accounting for only 12% of all valvular heart disease in Europe (compared to AS: 43%). Since 85% of cases follow rheumatic fever, there is wide geographical variation in incidence and prevalence, with up to 100 cases/100,000 population in India and as few as 1 case/100,000 population in the US.

Women seem more susceptible: MS is 2–3 times more common than in men, despite equivalent rates of rheumatic fever following streptococcal infection.

Aetiology

The vast majority of cases (85%) follow rheumatic fever. Other conditions (e.g. systemic lupus erythematosus, endomyocardial fibrosis) causing widespread inflammation can lead to MS. Congenital lesions are rare.

Rheumatic mitral stenosis

Group A haemolytic streptococcal pharyngeal infection results in rheumatic fever in 2–3% of patients. Autoimmune activation against the M protein antigen common to both the bacterium and the heart may result in pancarditis. Effects on the endocardium lead to valve inflammation and fibrosis. Predilection for the mitral valve is unexplained, but the combination of acute valve injury and ongoing low level inflammation leads to the classical lesion of rheumatic MS (Fig. 6.1).

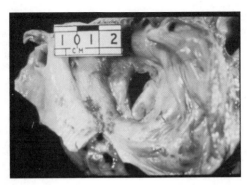

Fig. 6.1 Severe MS with thickening, fibrosis and fusion of commissures. See also **Plate 10**.

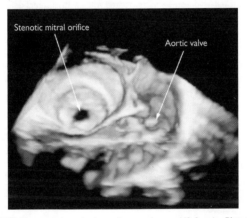

Fig. 6.2 3D Transoesophogeal echocardiogram of severe MS. See also **Plate 11**.

Other causes of mitral stenosis

Additional causes include mitral annular calcification (usually associated with AS), drugs (anorectic agents, e.g. fenfluramine–phentolamine, and methysergide), systemic lupus erythematosus, rheumatoid arthritis, and carcinoid syndrome. MS has also been reported in Hunter's syndrome (a rare mucopolysaccharidosis) and in eosinophilic fibroelastosis.

MS may also be mimicked by conditions causing mitral valve obstruction with a normal mitral valve (e.g. left atrial myxoma and left atrial ball thrombus).

Congenital mitral stenosis

Rare congenital lesions (annular hypoplasia, commissural fusion, and double orifice or parachute anatomy) can lead to MS but account for only 0.5% of all congenital heart disease (Fig. 6.3).

Congenital MS is often associated with other abnormalities (e.g. aortic coarctation and valvular or subvalvular AS). MS is a feature of Shone's syndrome (multiple left sided inflow and outflow obstructions including a supravalvular mitral membrane and parachute mitral valve) and Lutembacher's syndrome (MS associated with an atrial septal defect).

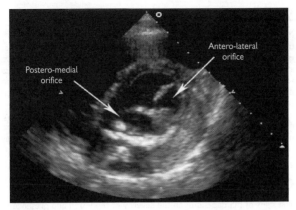

Fig. 6.3 Congenital double orifice mitral valve: the centres of the anterior and posterior leaflets are connected by a fibrous bridge resulting in two separate valve orifices.

Symptoms

Mitral valve area has to fall by around 50% (to approximately 2.5cm^2) before the onset of symptoms. Initially, cardiac output is maintained at rest but unable to increase sufficiently during exercise, emotional stress, infection, and pregnancy. Exertional dyspnoea and fatigue steadily progress to orthopnoea and paroxysmal nocturnal dyspnoea. Symptoms may then deteriorate abruptly with severe dyspnoea and pulmonary oedema, often related to the onset of atrial fibrillation.

Further (rarer) symptoms include haemoptysis (which can be significant if due to rupture of a dilated bronchial vein), dysphagia, lobar collapse, and hoarseness, all as a result of left atrial enlargement, chest pain, and other consequences of systemic embolism.

Clinical signs

The signs of MS depend upon the severity of the lesion and presence of associated complications. General findings include:
- Malar flush (mitral facies)
- Small volume pulse
- Atrial fibrillation
- V wave in JVP
- Tapping apex beat
- Palpable first heart sound
- Apical diastolic thrill
- Left parasternal heave (indicating RV hypertrophy).

Findings on auscultation include:
- Loud S1 (if sinus rhythm maintained)*
- Accentuated P2
- Opening snap (maximal in expiration at the apex)*
- Low pitched rumbling mid-diastolic murmur (maximal at the apex in the left lateral position)**
- Early diastolic murmur of PR (Graham–Steel murmur).

* Only present if valve is pliable.
** With pre-systolic accentuation if sinus rhythm is maintained. Progressing severity of MS is asso-ciated with abbreviation of the time interval between S2 and the opening snap, and prolongation of the diastolic murmur.

Complications

Complications result from the overall impact on cardiac function and secondary anatomical and functional changes:
• Left atrial enlargement (Fig. 6.4)
• Atrial fibrillation
• Systemic embolism
• Pulmonary hypertension
• TR
• RV failure
• Oesophageal compression
• Left recurrent laryngeal nerve palsy (Ortner's syndrome)
• Left main bronchus compression.

Natural history

The average age at presentation is between 40–50 years of age. One third of patients undergoing balloon mitral valvuloplasty are aged >65 years.

Serial assessment suggests a progressive fall in valve area of 0.1-0.3cm^2/year. A long asymptomatic period is associated with good prognosis and 80% ten year survival. Prognosis deteriorates dramatically once symptoms develop—mean survival with pulmonary hypertension is <3 years.

Left untreated, severe MS typically leads to death from pulmonary hypertension, systemic or pulmonary embolism, or infection.

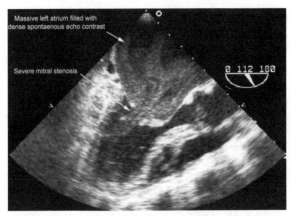

Fig. 6.4 Transoesophogeal echocardiogram of a massively dilated left atrium filled with spontaneous echo contrast due to severe mitral stenosis.

Initial investigations

Typical signs of MS in a breathless patient are usually sufficient for diagnosis. The ECG and chest X-ray may be helpful in patients with atrial fibrillation and/or low cardiac output when physical signs may be difficult to detect. Diagnosis is generally confirmed with echocardiography.

ECG

There are no diagnostic changes but the following may be seen (Fig. 6.5):
- Bifid P waves (if sinus rhythm is maintained) due to left atrial enlargement (P mitrale)
- Tall peaked P waves in pulmonary hypertension
- Right axis deviation and RBBB indicative of RV enlargement
- Atrial fibrillation.

Chest X-ray

The major findings are left atrial enlargement (Fig. 6.6) and pulmonary congestion:
- Straight left heart border
- Upper lobe venous diversion
- Pulmonary arterial dilation
- Double shadow of the left atrial border.

Differential diagnosis

Patients typically present with symptoms of heart failure and the main differential to consider is impaired LV function. Alternative diagnoses include:
- TS—usually associated with MS although right heart failure is predominant
- Atrial septal defect—fixed splitting of S2 and characteristic ECG changes
- Atrial myxoma.

MS should also be considered in all patients presenting with atrial fibrillation or systemic embolism.

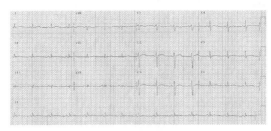

Fig. 6.5 ECG showing bifid P wave in lead II and biphasic P wave in V1, compatible with left atrial enlargement.

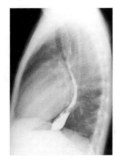

Fig. 6.6 Lateral chest X-ray during barium swallow showing oesophageal compression as a result of left atrial enlargement.

Echocardiographic assessment

Transthoracic echocardiography is the principal diagnostic investigation, allowing assessment of valve anatomy, overall cardiac function, potential complications, concomitant valve lesions and suitability for balloon mitral valvuloplasty. Transoesophageal echocardiography is usually undertaken as a secondary investigation, particularly when intervention is being considered.

Valve morphology

Classical findings in MS are restricted opening of the mitral valve leaflets with doming of the anterior leaflet leading to a typical 'hockey stick' configuration in the parasternal long axis view (Fig. 6.7).

In addition to leaflet mobility, the following should be carefully assessed:
- Leaflet thickness and flexibility
- Leaflet calcification
- Subvalvular fusion
- Commissural fusion
- Annular calcification.

Valve area

The severity of MS is assessed by measurement of valve area, either directly, or indirectly using Doppler flow measurements.

Direct planimetry is achieved by imaging the tips of the mitral valve in a parasternal short axis frame and tracing around the maximal orifice area (Fig. 6.8).

Doppler assessment

The severity of MS can be assessed by measurement of the pressure gradient across the valve. Using this information the valve area can be calculated based on the rate of decay of the gradient (Fig. 6.9).

Both peak and mean pressure gradient are measured by tracing around the spectral Doppler envelope of a continuous wave sample taken through the leaflet tips. Pressure half time is the time taken for peak gradient to fall to half of its maximal value. The valve area determined using the equation:

Mitral value area = 220/pressure half time (ms)

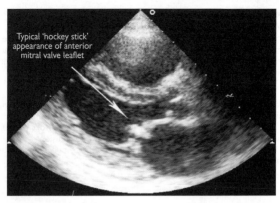

Fig. 6.7 Parasternal long axis image in diastole showing thickened mitral valve leaflets with calcified tips and doming of the anterior leaflet.

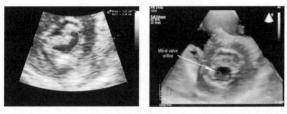

Fig. 6.8 Left hand panel: 2D planimetry from a parasternal short axis view zoomed onto the mitral valve orifice. The valve area is traced directly and appears elliptical in this patient. Right hand panel: corresponding 3D transthoracic view taken from a different patient.

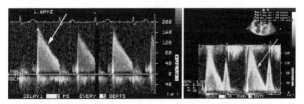

Fig. 6.9 The mean mitral valve gradient has been calculated by tracing around the trans-mitral Doppler signal (left hand panel, arrowed). The pressure half time may be estimated by tracing the mitral inflow deceleration slope (right hand panel).

Left ventricular size and function

LV cavity dimensions and overall systolic function are assessed in the standard manner. In the absence of any other valve pathology, the ventricle is usually small in size with normal systolic function. Dilation and impairment without coexistent coronary artery disease suggest persisting damage following myocarditis at the time of original rheumatic fever.

Associated abnormalities

Marked left atrial enlargement is common and may be associated with thrombus, particularly in a patient with atrial fibrillation (Fig. 6.10).

The presence of TR allows measurement of peak RV systolic pressure indicating the presence or absence of pulmonary hypertension.

Coexistent MR should be assessed using 2D colour Doppler and quantitative techniques.

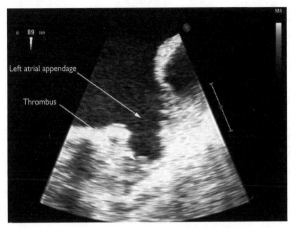

Fig. 6.10 Transoesophogeal echocardiogram of thrombus in a left atrial appendage in a patient with mitral stenosis and atrial fibrillation.

Grading severity

Severity of MS is graded according to a composite assessment of valve area, mean trans-valvar pressure gradient; pressure half time, symptomatic status, and the presence of pulmonary hypertension. No one single factor should be used in isolation.

Severity	Valve area (cm²)	Mean gradient (mmHg)	Pressure half time (ms)	Pulmonary pressure (mmHg)	Symptoms
Mild	2.2–1.5	2–4	100–150	<30	None
Moderate	1.2–1.5	4–9	150–180	<30	Class II
Moderate-severe	1.0–1.2	10–15	180–220	30–50	Class II–III
Severe	<1.0	>15	>220	>50	Class II–IV

Pitfalls

There are a number of potential confounders and care is required:

• The pressure half time equation assumes normal LV filling compliance and end-diastolic pressure. If either is elevated, for example in AR, the pressure gradient across the mitral valve will equalize more rapidly with resultant overestimation of valve area
• Atrial shunting will overestimate valve area if there is left to right flow—the converse is true if flow is in the opposite direction
• Atrial fibrillation will lead to variable filling time thereby affecting the pressure gradient—a mean should be determined over 2–3 cycles
• Impaired opening of the anterior mitral valve leaflet in significant AR can lead to underestimation of valve area
• Pressure half time assessment is sensitive to Doppler alignment—care must be taken to ensure that true peak velocity is recorded.

Avoiding assessment error

Ensure the following points are addressed:
- Accurate alignment of Doppler beam and flow through the mitral valve
- Average over 2–3 beats in atrial fibrillation
- Potential effects of concomitant AR or MR
- Potential effects of mitral annular calcification
- Exclude an atrial septal defect.

Transthoracic vs. transoesophageal echocardiography

MS can be reliably assessed with transthoracic echocardiography in the majority of patients—if acoustic windows are limited, a transoesophageal study will be required.

Transoesophageal echocardiography has superior sensitivity for the detection of left atrial appendage thrombus (99% vs. <50%) and should be performed if this is suspected.

If the findings of transthoracic echocardiography fail to correlate with the apparent severity of MS (e.g. significant pulmonary hypertension but only moderate MS) then transoesophageal imaging is warranted to ensure that significant MR has not been overlooked.

Transoesophageal echocardiography is undertaken in all patients in whom intervention is being considered to assess suitability for balloon mitral valvuloplasty or surgery.

Suitability for balloon mitral valvuloplasty

The suitability of the mitral valve for balloon valvuloplasty is determined by:
- Leaflet mobility
- Subvalvular thickening—including chordae and papillary muscles
- Leaflet thickness
- Leaflet calcification.

and exclusion of contraindications:
- Left atrial thrombus
- Moderate or severe MR
- Severe aortic valve disease
- Severe tricuspid valve disease.

Using these parameters, the Wilkins' score can be determined:

Grade	Mobility	Subvalvular thickening	Leaflet thickening	Leaflet calcification
1	Restricted tips only	Minimal thickening	Near normal thickness (4 – 5mm)	Single area of echo brightness
2	Reduced mobility at mid portion and base of leaflets	Thickening extending to 1/3 chordal length	Mild thickening	Scattered areas of brightness confined to leaflet margins
3	Valve leaflets move mainly at base	Thickening to distal third of chordae	Thickening through entire leaflet (5 – 8mm)	Brightness extending to mid portion of leaflets
4	Minimal leaflet movement	Thickening and shortening of all chordae	Marked thickening of whole leaflet (8 – 10mm)	Extensive brightness through whole leaflet

A score >8 suggests the likelihood of a poor immediate and long term result following balloon valvuloplasty (Fig. 6.11).

Additional imaging

The combination of transthoracic and transoesophageal echocardiography is sufficient in the vast majority of patients and further imaging is seldom required.

Ventricular dilation and impairment of no apparent cause can be further evaluated using CMR with late gadolinium enhancement and may demonstrate changes of previous myocarditis.

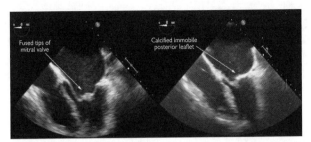

Fig. 6.11 The left hand panel shows a mitral valve suitable for valvuloplasty (Wilkins' score 4). The right hand panel shows a valve with less favourable features, notably the calcified and restricted posterior mitral valve leaflet (Wilkins' score >10).

Invasive assessment

Cardiac catheterization is still required in occasional patients where echocardiographic findings are inconclusive or correlate poorly with clinical symptoms and signs.

The following information may be obtained:
- Coronary anatomy
- Pulmonary capillary wedge pressure—surrogate for left atrial pressure
- Cardiac output
- Trans-valvar pressure gradient—using simultaneous measurement of left atrial and LV pressure
- Valve area (using Gorlin formula)
- Pulmonary artery pressure
- RV pressure
- Left ventriculography to assess systolic function and coexistent MR.

Direct measurement of left atrial pressure via trans-septal puncture is also feasible but rarely required.

Medical therapy

Asymptomatic patients in sinus rhythm require no specific treatment. Those with an embolic event or evidence of left atrial thrombus require anticoagulation with warfarin (or other vitamin K antagonist).

Atrial fibrillation is a common complication and often leads to abrupt symptomatic deterioration. Control of the ventricular rate using β blockers, rate limiting calcium channel antagonists, e.g. verapamil, or digoxin is required. Unstable patients with new onset atrial fibrillation may require electrical cardioversion.

The combination of atrial fibrillation and MS is associated with high embolic risk—around 10–15% per year. Anticoagulation is mandatory unless there are major contraindications. Pulmonary congestion and/or fluid overload respond well to regular diuretic therapy.

General measures

Patients should be reassured regarding the good long term prognosis, and advised of the benefits of anticoagulation (where appropriate) and potential for sudden deterioration associated with onset of atrial fibrillation.

Regular symptom limited low level aerobic exercise is safe and should be encouraged.

Surveillance

General measures

Patients should be advised to report symptoms early to allow the opportunity for timely reassessment and intervention.

Serial review

Asymptomatic patients should be reviewed annually. Echocardiographic assessment is required should there be a change in physical signs or clinical status.

All symptomatic patients should be assessed and considered for either balloon valvuloplasty or surgical intervention.

Indications for intervention

Patients with symptoms and a valve area <1.5cm^2 should be considered for intervention.

The following patients should be considered for balloon valvuloplasty:
- Symptomatic patients with favourable valve anatomy
- Symptomatic patients with contraindications to surgery.

The procedure should also be considered in asymptomatic patients at high risk of thromboembolism or haemodynamic decline:
- Previous thromboembolism
- Dense spontaneous contrast in the left atrium
- Paroxysmal atrial fibrillation
- Pulmonary artery pressure >50mmHg
- Need for major non-cardiac surgery
- Early or intended pregnancy.

If balloon valvuloplasty is not feasible due to unfavourable anatomy then either open commissurotomy or mitral valve replacement should be considered.

Open commissurotomy is rarely performed nowadays, although success rates are high with 96% survival and 92% freedom from valve-related complications at 15 years.

Closed commissurotomy (undertaken on the beating heart via the left atrial appendage) is now only performed in developing countries where cardiopulmonary bypass is unavailable.

Surgical therapy

Open commissurotomy requires a sternotomy and full cardiopulmonary bypass. The left atrium is usually entered via a horizontal left atriotomy and both the anterolateral and posteromedial commissures divided under direct vision. The major advantage over closed commissurotomy is the ability to carefully decalcify the leaflet and separate fused chordae.

If commissurotomy is not an option, mitral valve replacement is performed in the standard manner. As in other settings, the choice of prosthesis depends on patient factors, including age, safety of anticoagulation, risk of re-do surgery and any pre-existent indications for lifelong anticoagulation (e.g. atrial fibrillation).

Balloon valvuloplasty for MS via a percutaneous approach is a long standing effective technique for the treatment of MS (see 📖 p.306).

Mitral stenosis and tricuspid regurgitation

Pathophysiology

The usual cause of TR in patients with MS is secondary changes of the tricuspid annulus and RV in response to pulmonary hypertension (Fig. 6.12). However, the rheumatic process responsible for almost all MS may also cause rheumatic changes to the tricuspid valve.

Management

The management strategy is directed towards the MS, and balloon mitral valvuloplasty may be the preferred option with subsequent monitoring of pulmonary pressure and TR.

In patients requiring mitral valve replacement for MS the decision whether to also operate on the tricuspid valve is often difficult. In cases of severe pulmonary hypertension but no overt tricuspid valve deformity, the TR is likely to improve with relief of left sided obstruction.

Conversely, a low threshold for tricuspid annuloplasty (Fig. 6.13) is reasonable if there is significant deformity of the valve or marked annular dilation. Replacement is occasionally necessary.

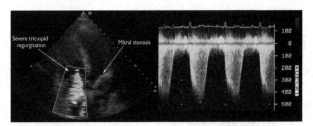

Fig. 6.12 Transthoracic echocardiogram demonstrating severe tricuspid regurgitation due to mitral stenosis induced pulmonary hypertension. See also **Plate 12.**

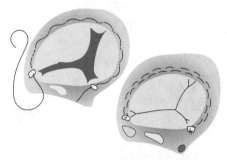

Fig. 6.13 Example of a classical De Vega style annuloplasty. Reproduced from Antunes M.J., Barlow J.B. (2007) Management of tricuspid valve regurgitation *Heart*; 93:271–276 with permission from BMJ Publishing Group Ltd.

Mitral stenosis and aortic stenosis

Pathophysiology

This combination is almost always due to rheumatic heart disease. As the effect of MS is to reduce LV filling and hence stroke volume the velocities and pressure drop across the aortic valve will be reduced leading to underestimation of severity.

This scenario is analogous to low-flow low-gradient AS (see 📖 p.121). However, dobutamine stress echocardiography is unhelpful given the deleterious effects of tachycardia on LV filling in MS. An important implication of this combination is that the aortic signs often dominate the clinical picture even if MS is the dominant lesion – careful assessment of the mitral valve is mandatory in all patients with AS.

Management

Management is directed at the dominant lesion – if the mitral valve is suitable then balloon mitral valvuloplasty should be undertaken, with subsequent re-assessment of the aortic valve following this. High risk patients could potentially be treated by balloon mitral valvuloplasty, followed by transcatheter aortic valve implantation when required (see 📖 p.314).

Mitral stenosis and aortic regurgitation

Pathophysiology

In this scenario the MS is usually severe and AR mild, the pathophysiology and clinical findings of MS being dominant. If the AR is severe this may not be easily apparent as LV dilation is reduced and clinical signs of AR will be less apparent.

AR increases LV diastolic pressure and reduces the gradient between the left atrium and LV, thereby leading to an underestimation of the severity of MS. Careful echocardiography and cardiac catheterization are usually required to fully assess this combination of lesions.

Management

Management may involve double valve replacement but a reasonable strategy in many patients is to perform initial balloon mitral valvuloplasty. This may relieve the dominant lesion with symptomatic improvement, allowing monitoring and deferred surgical treatment of the AR if required.

MS in patients needing CABG

Patients with moderate to severe MS who require CABG (or aortic valve replacement) should be considered for concomitant mitral valve surgery.

Selected patients with MS and aortic valve disease may benefit from initial balloon mitral valvuloplasty followed by aortic valve replacement to avoid the risks of double valve surgery. Similarly, initial balloon valvuloplasty may defer the need for surgery in a patient with severe MS and moderate aortic valve disease.

Management algorithm for severe mitral stenosis

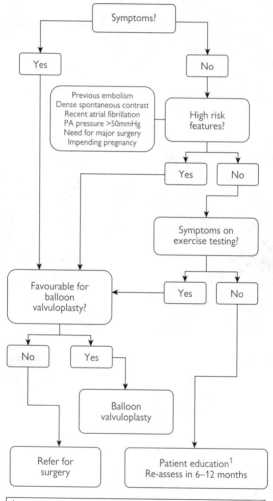

¹Advise on symptoms and need for early reporting

Mitral regurgitation

Introduction

MR is common and may result from abnormal function of any part of the mitral valve complex—the valve leaflets, annulus, chordae tendinae, and papillary muscles.

Acute MR is a medical emergency and high risk surgery is often necessary. In contrast, chronic MR is usually well tolerated: detailed assessment and follow up are required to optimize the timing of intervention and choice of surgical technique.

Epidemiology

MR is the most common valve lesion after AS, accounting for one third of all cases of valvular heart disease, and is now more common than MS in developed nations as a result of the decline of rheumatic fever.

The overall prevalence of significant MR is 12% in males and 13% in females, and increases with age: 5% in those >30 years and 17% in those >80 years.

Aetiology

MR may be due to a primary abnormality of the mitral valve complex or secondary to other cardiac disease.

Abnormalities of mitral valve complex

Disease of the leaflets, annulus, chordae or papillary muscles (in isolation or combination) can lead to MR—the most common cause is degenerative valvular heart disease with myxomatous leaflet degeneration.

Degenerative mitral valve disease

Mitral valve prolapse is common, may exist in isolation or in association with any degree of MR, and is usually caused by myxomatous degeneration. When identified in young patients with excess leaflet tissue, it is often termed Barlow's syndrome. In more elderly patients there is no excess leaflet tissue but fibroelastic deficiency. Characteristic changes include leaflet thickening, chordal elongation, and annular dilation due to alterations in extracellular matrix components (collagen, elastin, and matrix metalloproteinases). Most cases are sporadic but an autosomal dominant form (with variable penetrance) has been mapped to chromosomes 11 and 16. Definitions vary, but single or bileaflet prolapse at least 2mm beyond the long axis annular plane is a generally accepted cut-off. Applying these criteria, mitral valve prolapse can be identified in around 3% of the normal population (Fig. 7.1).

Mitral valve prolapse is more common in women but more men are referred for surgical intervention. It is unclear whether this represents referral bias or gender differences in the progression of disease or compensatory mechanisms.

Overall, up to 10% of patients with mitral valve prolapse will progress to severe MR. Left untreated the mortality rate is 7% per year.

Infective endocarditis

Bacterial proliferation and inflammation may result in leaflet erosion and/ or perforation. Large mobile vegetations may also disrupt leaflet co-aptation with resultant MR.

Rheumatic heart disease

Although rare in Western societies, rheumatic valvular heart disease remains an important cause of MR in developing nations. Whilst typically resulting in MS, up to one third of patients develop pure MR, often in the setting of uncontrolled carditis with rapid leaflet damage.

Many patients with MS have additional MR, the extent of which may limit the applicability of balloon valvuloplasty.

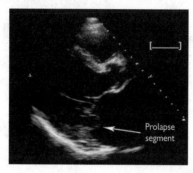

Prolapse
segment

Fig. 7.1 Prolapse of a posterior leaflet segment into the left atrium beyond the mitral annular plane.

Mitral valve prolapse with normal leaflets

Mitral valve prolapse may also be seen without leaflet thickening or evidence of myxomatous degeneration, usually as a result of abnormally long chordae or excess leaflet tissue. Reduced LV volumes may also lead to slackening of the papillary muscle/chordae with resultant valve prolapse.

Congenital abnormalities

Congenital MR is rare but can be due to:

- Anterior leaflet cleft with atrioventricular canal defect (Fig. 7.2)
- Isolated anterior leaflet cleft
- Posterior leaflet cleft—often with papillary muscle abnormalities
- Papillary muscle abnormalities (absent or deficient)
- Congenitally corrected transposition of the great arteries
- Double orifice mitral valve—usually with asymmetric orifices.

Connective tissue disease

Around 90% of patients with Marfan's syndrome have typical features of mitral valve prolapse as a result of altered LV geometry and abnormal valve tissue.

Mitral valve prolapse is much less common in other connective tissue disorders (~5% in Ehler's–Danlos syndrome).

Systemic lupus erythematosus

Libman–Sacks endocarditis may accompany the anti-phospholipid syndrome resulting in mitral valve thickening or non-infective vegetations. Valve lesions are usually minor and rarely clinically significant.

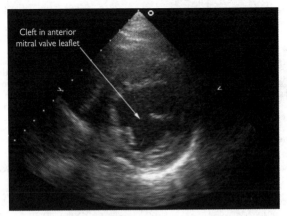

Fig. 7.2 Transthoracic echocardiogram of a cleft anterior mitral valve leaflet.

Secondary to cardiac disease

MR may arise without apparent abnormality of the valve leaflets or sub-valvar apparatus. Management options are crucially dependent on the underlying mechanism and accurate assessment is vital.

Functional MR arises due to abnormalities of the LV myocardium (including the papillary muscles) resulting in dilation of the mitral annulus. Common causes include dilated cardiomyopathy and ischaemic heart disease.

Ischaemic MR arises as a consequence of regional myocardial ischaemia or infarction with resultant papillary muscle or leaflet dysfunction.

In practice, the syndromes frequently overlap and a combined mechanism is observed in many patients.

Ischaemic mitral regurgitation

Acute ischaemic MR is usually a consequence of acute myocardial infarction with partial or complete papillary muscle rupture.

Chronic ischaemic MR arises as a result of changes in LV structure, geometry and function, usually in patients with long standing stable coronary artery disease or survivors of major myocardial infarction with associated extensive LV impairment.

Papillary muscle displacement due to abnormal remodelling of attached ventricular wall has two effects: displacement of the leaflets away from the usual closure line and an increase in the distance from the papillary muscles to the annulus. This change in tethering length and angle, along with reduced ventricular force to close the leaflets causes incomplete mitral valve closure and resultant MR (Fig. 7.3).

Another key aspect of ischaemic MR is the dynamic nature of the changes in geometry and function of the mitral valve complex. Apparently mild lesions at rest may become more significant with exercise induced ischaemia. Similarly, even moderate or severe MR may appear only mild once the patient is anaesthetized and vasodilated prior to surgery. Assessment must always take account of the prevailing haemodynamic status.

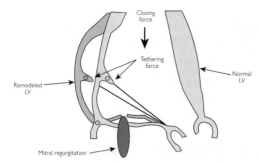

Fig. 7.3 Mechanism of ischaemic MR—papillary muscle displacement and leaflet tethering restricts leaflet closure. Reproduced from Agricola E., Oppizzi M., Pisani M. et al. (2008) *European Journal of Echocardiography* 9:207–221.

Functional mitral regurgitation

LV enlargement combined with altered geometry and annular dilation displaces the papillary muscles and reduces leaflet coaptation with resultant MR (Fig. 7.4).

Ventricular dyssynchrony as a result of left bundle branch block or RV apical pacing may have similar effects. Resynchronization using biventricular pacing can significantly reduce functional MR in selected patients.

Ischaemic vs. functional mitral regurgitation

The distinction between ischemic and functional MR is frequently difficult and overlap is common. The following pointers are helpful:

Ischaemic mitral regurgitation	Functional mitral regurgitation
Myocardial infarction with local remodelling (usually inferior wall)	Global LV abnormalities
Asymmetrical leaflet tethering—usually posterior	Symmetrical leaflet tethering—usually apical
Asymmetric regurgitant jet	Central symmetrical regurgitant jet
Annulus often normal	Annular dilation usually present

Hypertrophic cardiomyopathy

Asymmetric septal thickening is associated with a dynamic LV outflow tract gradient in classical hypertrophic cardiomyopathy. The high velocity jet draws the anterior mitral leaflet towards the septum in systole (systolic anterior motion, SAM). This displacement further increases outflow tract obstruction and affects leaflet co-aptation resulting in a posteriorly directed jet of mild to moderate MR.

Severe or anteriorly directed MR is unusual and should prompt a detailed search for additional valve pathology.

Other congenital lesions

Mitral valve prolapse is detected in two thirds of patients with a secundum atrial septal defect, usually as a result of a small and distorted LV. Repair of the atrial septal defect restores ventricular geometry and size with resolution of the prolapse in most cases.

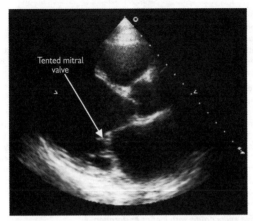

Fig. 7.4 Idiopathic dilated cardiomyopathy with severe LV dilation and marked tenting of the mitral valve (arrowed).

Causes of acute mitral regurgitation
• Papillary muscle rupture complicating acute myocardial infarction.
• IE with leaflet perforation.
• Traumatic damage to chordae or leaflets (e.g. balloon valvuloplasty).
• Flail leaflet or chordal rupture complicating degenerative valvular heart disease.

Papillary muscle rupture
Sudden partial or complete rupture of a papillary muscle is a rare complication, typically arising 2–7 days after acute myocardial infarction. The posteromedial papillary muscle receives a single blood supply from the posterior descending artery and is more frequently involved (75%). The anterolateral papillary muscle typically receives its blood supply from both the diagonal (LAD) and marginal (circumflex) and has less mechanical stress due to its superior location relative to the annulus. Papillary muscle rupture is also more common in patients with single vessel disease due to the absence of a collateral blood supply. Acute papillary muscle rupture leads to a flail leaflet(s) and sudden torrential MR.

Infective endocarditis with leaflet perforation
IE typically leads to vegetation formation which may result in valve disruption and regurgitation. Aggressive organisms, e.g. *Staphylococcus aureus*, may cause abscess formation, leaflet destruction, and perforation.

Traumatic damage
Direct valvular trauma during cardiac instrumentation or catheterization can lead to chordal rupture and flail leaflet.

Balloon mitral valvuloplasty (see 📖 p.306) is associated with a small risk (2–10%) of traumatic damage to the thickened leaflets and chordae, causing a flail leaflet and severe MR requiring immediate surgery.

Flail leaflet in degenerative mitral valve disease
Leaflet prolapse and elongated chordae are common—superimposed chordal rupture may result in a flail segment with associated abrupt severe MR (Fig. 7.5).

Causes of chronic mitral regurgitation

Abnormalities of the mitral valve complex:
- Degenerative valvular heart disease
- Mitral valve prolapse
- IE
- Rheumatic heart disease
- Congenital valve abnormality
- Drugs (e.g. ergotamine and cabergoline)
- Trauma with chordal or papillary muscle rupture
- Connective tissue disease (Marfan's syndrome, Ehler's–Danlos syndrome, osteogenesis imperfecta, pseudoxanthoma elasticum, psoriatic arthritis, systemic lupus erythematosus).

Secondary to other cardiac disease:
- Ischaemic heart disease—'ischaemic MR'
- LV dilation—'functional MR'
- Hypertrophic cardiomyopathy
- Other congenital lesions.

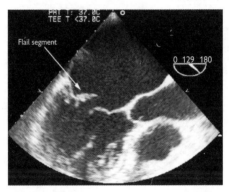

Fig. 7.5 Flail segment of posterior mitral valve leaflet (arrowed) complicating degenerative mitral valve disease.

Symptoms

Factors influencing the development of symptoms in MR include:
- Severity of regurgitation
- Rate of onset
- Rate of progression
- Pulmonary hypertension
- Additional valve or ventricular disease.

Acute severe MR presents with sudden severe pulmonary oedema.

Chronic MR typically remains asymptomatic for many years before presentation with dyspnoea, fatigue, and weakness as a result of an inadequate rise in cardiac output during exertion. Palpitations may relate to the development of atrial fibrillation.

Further decompensation may produce symptoms of heart failure during mild exertion or episodes of pulmonary oedema during concurrent illness or stress. Right sided heart failure as a consequence of pulmonary hypertension may be seen in end-stage disease.

Asymptomatic patients may also present with complications of their mitral valve disease, e.g. IE.

Mitral valve prolapse has been associated with a variety of symptoms including:
- Palpitations
- Syncope
- Anxiety disorder
- Exercise intolerance
- Chest pain
- Hyperventilation.

The pathophysiology of these symptoms may relate to neuroendocrine or autonomic dysfunction and is poorly understood. Treatment options are limited.

Clinical signs

Clinical signs depend on the severity of the MR and degree of decompensation:
- Brisk arterial upstroke—due to reduced afterload and increased stroke volume
- Normal pulse pressure
- Hyperdynamic displaced apex—dilated vigorous LV
- Palpable thrill—in severe MR
- Diminished 1st heart sound and split second heart sound
- Audible third heart sound—common
- Palpable third heart sound—rapid LV filling in early diastole.

The murmur of MR is variable and depends on the aetiology, severity, and direction of the regurgitant jet. Assessment based upon this alone is of limited accuracy. The classical murmur is typically pansystolic (loudest at the apex radiating to the axilla and back) with a blowing high pitched quality.

Common variations include:
- Murmur loudest at base—jet directed anteriorly towards the aortic root due to posterior leaflet pathology
- Murmur loudest at the back—jet directed posteriorly due to anterior leaflet pathology
- Mid systolic click relating to mitral valve prolapse
- Short late systolic murmur—associated with mitral valve prolapse or papillary muscle dysfunction.

Signs of RV dysfunction are rare unless there is additional MS or pulmonary hypertension.

Complications

The principal complication is LV failure as a consequence of increased workload and cardiac dilation.

Additional complications include:
- Atrial and ventricular ectopy—extremely common
- Atrial fibrillation—5%/year
- Systemic embolism due to left atrial thrombus—overall risk is low
- IE—<1% over 5 years
- Sudden cardiac death—rare but more likely if severe MR or flail leaflet.

Natural history

The natural history of MR is clearly dependent on its aetiology.

Ten year longitudinal data in patients with classical mitral valve prolapse in the USA suggest:
- Overall survival 81%
- Freedom from cardiovascular mortality 91%
- Cardiovascular morbidity 30%
- Complications 20%
- Mitral valve replacement 8%.

Factors predicting cardiovascular mortality include:
- Moderate to severe MR
- LV ejection fraction <50%
- Left atrial dimension >40mm
- Flail leaflet
- Atrial fibrillation
- Age >50 years.

(Avierinos J.F., Gersh B.J., Melton L.J. et al. (2002) Circulation 106:1355–1361)

Initial investigations

Diagnosis is usually suspected on the basis of an abnormal clinical examination and confirmed with echocardiography. However, additional information may be helpful in the identification of complications and assessment of risk.

ECG

There are no specific ECG changes in MR but abnormalities relating to structural changes of the left atrium and LV may be seen:
- Left atrial enlargement—broad P wave in lead II, biphasic in V1
- LV hypertrophy
- RV hypertrophy in pulmonary hypertension.

Ventricular ectopics are common and atrial fibrillation may be associated with left atrial enlargement.

Chest X-ray

The most likely abnormality is enlargement of the cardiac silhouette due to LV dilation. Additional changes include:
- Globular cardiac silhouette—large spherical LV
- Left atrial enlargement—straightened left heart border
- Left main bronchus displaced superiorly
- Mitral annular calcification—rare in isolated MR
- Pulmonary oedema—in congestive heart failure
- Pulmonary arterial enlargement—in pulmonary hypertension.

Differential diagnosis

Additional causes of a pansystolic murmur in an asymptomatic patient include:
- TR—murmur increases on inspiration, abnormal JVP
- VSD—murmur usually radiates to right sternal edge.

Echocardiographic assessment

Echocardiography is the best investigation for identification of the pathology of MR and grading severity. Careful assessment of the entire mitral valve complex and the LV is required to clarify the abnormalities and guide management.

Valve morphology

The valve leaflets should be imaged in multiple planes to ensure all aspects have been visualized. The following details should be assessed:
- Leaflet thickness
- Leaflet mobility
- Leaflet calcification
- Leaflet prolapse—>2mm tip excursion beyond the annular plane
- Masses or vegetations
- Flail segments or ruptured chordae.

Mitral annulus

The annulus is best imaged and measured in the parasternal long-axis and apical 4-chamber views. Three-dimensional assessment is of particular value and allows planning of surgery, where applicable. The following details should be assessed:
- Annular diameter in two orthogonal planes
- Calcification
- Annular bulging/displacement with wall motion abnormalities.

Papillary muscles

The papillary muscles and major chordae are readily identified using transthoracic echocardiography. Their position, size, shape, and appearance should be assessed.

Congenital abnormalities of the papillary muscle positions are rare.

Left ventricle

LV systolic and diastolic diameters are measured in the parasternal long-axis view and ejection fraction calculated using the bi-plane disc method or 3D quantification.

Additional information required includes:
- Shape and sphericity
- Global or regional wall motion abnormalities
- Presence/absence of aneurysm.

Dyssynchrony

Disorganized contraction of the LV can cause or exacerbate MR—assessment for the presence or absence of dyssynchrony should be undertaken as required.

Carpentier classification

Once complete assessment of the mitral valve complex has been performed, the mechanism of MR can be categorized:

Carpentier type I (Fig. 7.6)

Normal leaflet motion with no prolapse—MR is usually due to:

- Annular dilation
- Leaflet perforation.

Carpentier type II (Fig. 7.7)

Abnormal leaflet motion with one or more leaflets passing into the left atrium beyond the annular plane—MR is usually due to:

- Leaflet prolapse
- Chordal rupture
- Chordal elongation
- Papillary muscle rupture.

Carpentier type III (Fig. 7.8)

Restricted leaflet motion with incomplete return to the closure point:

- Type IIIa—valvular or subvalvular thickening (usually due to rheumatic disease)
- Type IIIb—papillary muscle displacement and tethering (usually due to ischaemic remodelling, papillary muscle displacement or functional MR in global LV dilation).

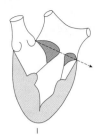

Fig. 7.6 Carpentier type I lesion—normal leaflet motion.

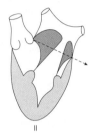

Fig. 7.7 Carpentier type II lesion—leaflets pass beyond the annular plane (dashed line).

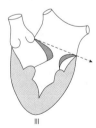

Fig. 7.8 Carpentier type III—restricted leaflet motion.

Doppler assessment

Numerous parameters can be used in the assessment of MR:
• Colour Doppler jet area
• Vena contracta width
• Flow convergence (PISA)
• Mitral valve inflow
• Pulmonary vein Doppler
• Regurgitant volume.

All have potential pitfalls and care must be taken to ensure optimal image settings. No one parameter is perfect and combined quantitative and qualitative assessment is required.

Colour Doppler jet area

The most basic assessment is derived by colour Doppler sampling in the left atrium. Imaging in multiple views allows assessment of:
• Jet direction (anterior jet = posterior leaflet pathology and *vice versa*)
• Jet area relative to the size of the left atrium
• Mechanism of regurgitation—central or through leaflet perforation
• Jet eccentricity—e.g. entrainment along the atrial wall
• Multiple jets.

The size of the regurgitant jet provides a guide to severity (Fig. 7.9) but requires integration with additional parameters (including quantitative assessment where possible).

Potential pitfalls include:
• Incorrect settings: lower sampling limit (overestimates MR)
• Entrainment of left atrial blood into the jet (underestimates MR)
• Eccentric jets (underestimates MR, the Coanda effect)
• Jets which flow out of the imaging plane (underestimates MR).

Vena contracta

Measurement of the diameter of the narrowest portion of the regurgitant jet allows derivation of the regurgitant orifice area. The measurement is small (usually <1cm, even in severe MR), easily affected by colour gain settings and image resolution, and therefore prone to error.

Other pitfalls include:
• Multiple jets underestimate MR
• Limited resolution of lateral plane—use parasternal window if possible
• Irregular jet shape—the regurgitant orifice is rarely circular
• Atrial fibrillation—beat to beat variation in regurgitant volume
• Dynamic orifice—may vary in size during systole.

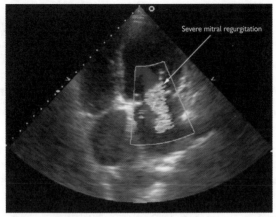

Fig. 7.9 Transthoracic echocardiogram demonstrating severe MR: the broad colour jet occupies at least 2/3 of the left atrium. See also **Plate 13.**

Flow convergence

Measurement of the PISA (see 📖 p.64) can be used to derive the regurgitant flow, EROA, and regurgitant volume. The jet is imaged in the long axis (apical 4-chamber for transthoracic echocardiography) and the colour jet image optimized. The colour Doppler baseline (not the scale) is then adjusted in the direction of the regurgitant jet (down in transthoracic, up in transoesophageal) to usually a Nyquist limit of around 40cm/s. The image is further optimized and zoomed until a clear arc of flow convergence is identified. The radius of this arc is then measured from a still frame (Fig. 7.10).

$PISA$ (regurgitant flow) $= 2\pi \times r^2 \times$ aliasing velocity

$EROA = PISA/$peak regurgitant velocity*

Regurgitant volume $= EROA \times$ Regurgitation VTI*

Mitral valve inflow

The velocity of flow across the mitral valve during diastole is increased in MR as a result of the increased atrioventricular pressure gradient and can be measured using pulsed wave Doppler (Fig. 7.11).

Potential pitfalls include:
• Effects of preload
• Associated MS (increased E wave)
• Hyperdynamic circulation (increased E wave).

Mitral inflow pattern and E wave velocity is only a crude guide to the severity of regurgitation. However, severe MR is very unlikely if the A wave is dominant.

Pulmonary vein Doppler

The pulmonary veins normally provide continuous inflow into the left atrium (other than brief flow reversal during atrial systole). This flow is attenuated in MR as a result of rising left atrial pressure and may actually be reversed during systole in severe MR (Fig. 7.12).

Potential pitfalls include:
• Limited pulmonary vein imaging with transthoracic echocardiography
• Attenuation of pulmonary vein systolic flow is a non-specific finding in all causes of raised left atrial pressure
• Eccentric MR may not cause flow reversal in all four pulmonary veins.

---

* Derived from continuous wave Doppler aligned with regurgitant jet.

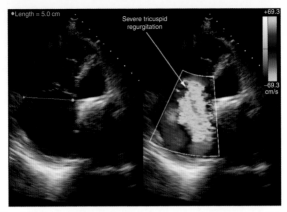

Plate 1 (Fig. 1.16) Transthoracic echocardiogram demonstrating a severely dilated right ventricle with tricuspid regurgitation due to dilation of the tricuspid annulus.

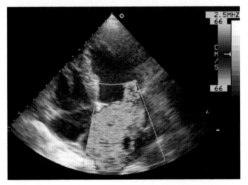

Plate 2 (Fig. 2.9) Colour flow mapping of MR. Note the large 'blue flame' of regurgitation.

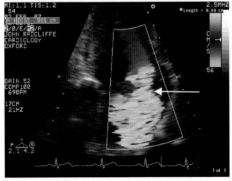

Plate 3 (Fig. 2.14) Zoomed view of MR using colour flow mapping to demonstrate the vena contracta (arrowed).

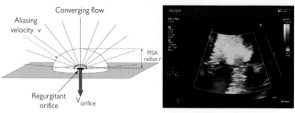

Plate 4 (Fig. 2.15) The left hand panel is a schematic representation of PISA measurement. The right hand panel is a colour flow image showing the hemispheric 'shell' of flow convergence. The colour scale baseline has been altered so that a clear hemisphere of flow at a single velocity is seen, identified by transition of the colour jet (from blue to yellow, arrowed) at the limit of the velocity range
Left hand panel reproduced from Irvine T., Li XK, Sahn D.J., Kenny A. (2002) Assessment of mitral regurgitation *Heart*; 88:11–19 with permission from BMJ Publishing Group Ltd.

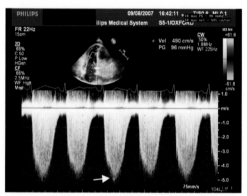

Plate 5 (Fig. 2.18) Continuous wave Doppler of TR. The peak velocity of 5m/s (arrowed) suggests a peak pressure drop of 100mmHg indicating severe pulmonary hypertension.

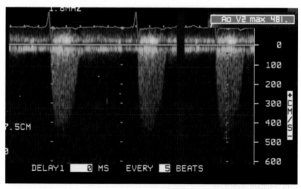

Plate 6 (Fig. 4.6) Continuous wave Doppler in severe aortic stenosis—peak velocity nearly 5m/s.

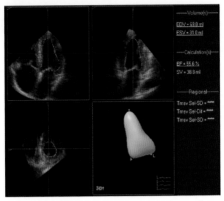

Plate 7 (Fig. 5.6) Three-dimensional assessment of LV volume and ejection fraction. If accurate determination of ejection fraction is not possible using echocardiography then radionuclide ventriculography or cardiac magnetic resonance imaging provide a valid alternative.

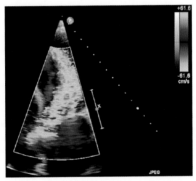

Plate 8 (Fig. 5.7) Apical 5-chamber view demonstrating a wide jet of severe AR in the LV outflow tract extending to the apex.

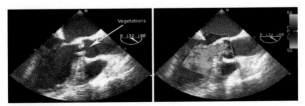

Plate 9 (Fig. 5.10) Transoesophageal echocardiogram in aortic valve IE demonstrating large vegetations on both the non-coronary and right-coronary cusps. A diastolic image (left hand panel) shows a clear defect in the valve (arrowed) with resultant severe AR (right hand panel)—the colour flow signal occupies the entire LV outflow tract.

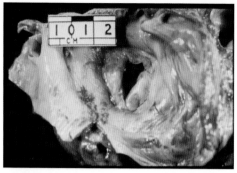

Plate 10 (Fig. 6.1) Severe MS with thickening, fibrosis and fusion of commissures.

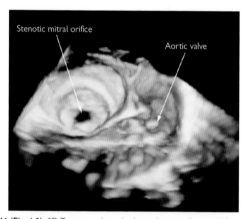

Plate 11 (Fig. 6.2) 3D Transoesophogeal echocardiogram of severe MS.

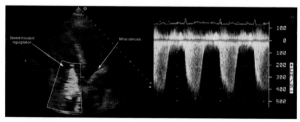

Plate 12 (Fig. 6.12) Transthoracic echocardiogram demonstrating severe tricuspid regurgitation due to mitral stenosis induced pulmonary hypertension.

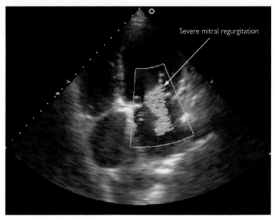

Plate 13 (Fig. 7.9) Transthoracic echocardiogram demonstrating severe MR: the broad colour jet occupies at least 2/3 of the left atrium.

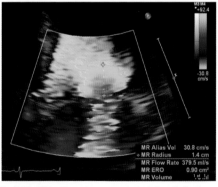

Plate 14 (Fig. 7.10) PISA with semi-automated calculation of effective regurgitant orifice area and regurgitant volume.

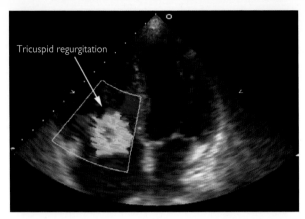

Plate 15 (Fig. 9.2) A very broad jet of TR on colour flow Doppler—the tricuspid leaflets are fixed in an open position due to carcinoid disease.

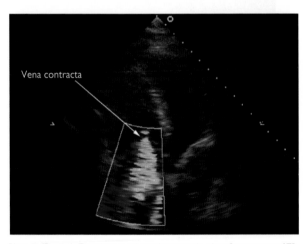

Plate 16 (Fig. 9.6) Transthoracic echocardiogram with colour flow mapping of TR demonstrating the vena contracta.

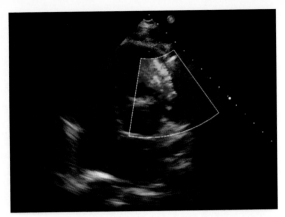

Plate 17 (Fig. 11.1) Pulmonary regurgitation demonstrated on echocardiography in a patient with previous pulmonary valve replacement with a homograft.

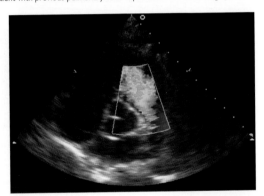

Plate 18 (Fig. 11.3) Colour flow Doppler demonstrating a broad jet of pulmonary regurgitation.

A B

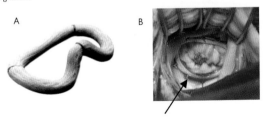

Plate 19 (Fig. 12.6) (a) Edwards Geoform ring (B) implanted annuloplasty ring. From Edwards Lifesciences website
 http://www.edwards.com/products/rings/geoform.htm and ESC website
 http://www.escardio.org/communities/councils/ccp/e-journal/volume7/pages/ infective-endocarditis.aspx respectively.

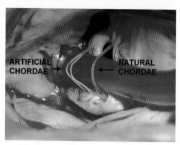

ARTIFICIAL CHORDAE → ← NATURAL CHORDAE

Plate 20 (Fig. 12.7) Surgically implanted artificial chordae with natural chordae alongside for comparison. From website ℘ http://www.westernthoracic.org/Abstracts/2007/9.html.

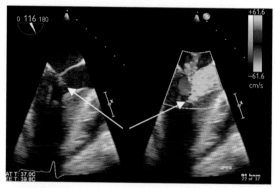

Plate 21 (Fig.12.9) Postoperative SAM—the anterior leaflet deviates into the outflow tract during systole with resultant flow obstruction (highlighted with colour Doppler—arrowed). These changes resolved with increased filling pressures and reduced inotropic support.

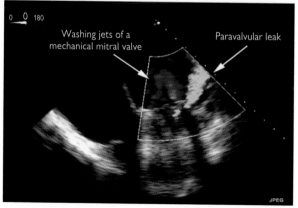

Washing jets of a mechanical mitral valve   Paravalvular leak

Plate 22 (Fig. 12.12) Transoesophogeal echocardiogram of a paraprosthetic leak—this narrow high velocity jet was causing persistent haemolysis.

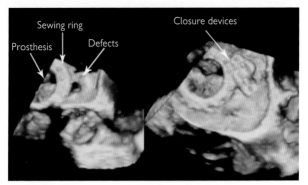

Plate 23 (Fig. 12.13) 3D transoesophageal imaging. The left hand panel shows a mitral bioprosthesis with two defects around the sewing ring. The right hand panel demonstrates the final appearance of two occluder devices deployed across the defect to abolish the MR.

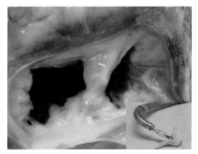

Plate 24 (Fig. 13.4) Results 6 months after deployment of an Evalve clip in a porcine model.
Reproduced from Coats, Bonhoeffer (2007) New percutaneous treatments for heart disease, *Heart*; 93:639–644) with permission of BMJ Publishing Group Ltd.

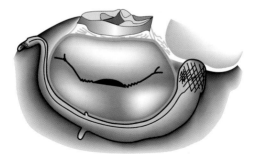

Plate 25 (Fig.13.5) The Edwards Monarch system—a shaped constraining device deployed in the coronary sinus.

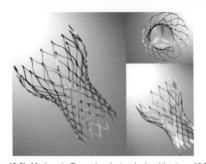

Plate 26 (Fig. 13.8) Medtronic Corevalve device deployable via an 18 French delivery system.
Taken from ✍ www.edwards.com/products/transcathetervalves/sapienthv.htm

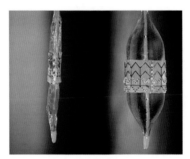

Plate 27 (Fig. 13.9) The Edwards Sapien valve.
Taken from ✍ http://www.edwards.com/products/transcathetervalves/sapienthv.htm.

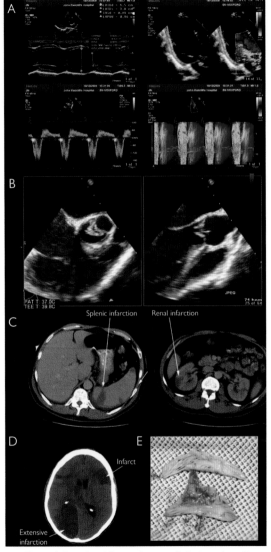

Plate 28 (Fig. 16.1) Examples of the complications of infective endocarditis.

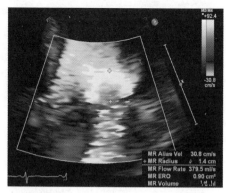

Fig. 7.10 PISA with semi-automated calculation of effective regurgitant orifice area and regurgitant volume. See also **Plate 14**.

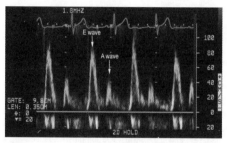

Fig. 7.11 Pulsed wave Doppler at the mitral leaflet tips demonstrating passive ventricular filling (E wave) and atrial systole (A wave occurring after P wave on ECG).

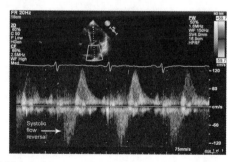

Fig. 7.12 Marked pulmonary vein systolic flow reversal in severe MR.

Regurgitant volume

In the absence of MR, the volume of blood crossing the mitral valve into the LV in diastole should equal the volume entering the aorta during systole (assuming no shunts or AR).

Mitral inflow volume is derived by measuring the VTI at valve level and estimating valve area from the annular diameter:

Mitral inflow volume = mitral valve VTI x area

Aortic outflow volume is derived by measuring VTI in the LVOT and the LVOT cross sectional area:

LV outflow volume = LVOT VTI x area

Regurgitant volume and fraction can then be calculated:

Regurgitant volume = Mitral inflow volume − LV outflow volume

Regurgitant fraction = Mitral regurgitant volume/mitral inflow volume

As previously described regurgitant orifice area can also be derived from the PISA method:

EROA = regurgitant volume/VTI of MR jet

Potential pitfalls include:
- Difficulties measuring annular diameter—any errors are squared
- Particular difficulties in presence of mitral annular calcification
- Overestimating mitral velocity jet
- Inaccurate volume sample placement
- Time consuming measurements and calculations
- Inaccurate in the presence of associated AR.

Left ventricular size and function

LV shape and dimensions in end-systole and end-diastole should be carefully assessed, and the mitral valve annulus measured in two planes (Fig. 7.13).

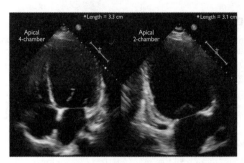

Fig. 7.13 Measurement of the mitral valve annulus in both the apical 4-chamber and 2-chamber views.

Associated abnormalities

The following should be assessed, particularly if intervention is contemplated:
- Abnormalities of RV size and function
- Pulmonary arterial systolic pressure
- Left atrial size and volume
- Left atrial appendage thrombus.

Advanced assessment using tissue Doppler interrogation and strain imaging may assist the identification of impaired ventricles with normal ejection fraction.

Transthoracic vs. transoesophageal echocardiography

Transoesophageal echocardiography is not mandatory in the assessment of MR but should be strongly considered in the following situations:
- Transthoracic assessment inconsistent with clinical picture
- Unclear mechanism of MR
- Suspected IE
- Prior to valve repair
- Patients with at least mild MR undergoing other cardiac surgery.

Grading severity

Assessment of the severity of MR is best achieved by integration of all available measurements—no method alone is sufficiently robust for accurate grading.

	Mild	Moderate	Severe
Jet area (Nyquist 50–60cm/s)	<4cm^2 <20% of the left atrium	Variable	>10cm^2 >40% of the left atrium
Vena contracta	<0.3cm	0.3–0.7cm	>0.7cm
PISA radius (Nyquist 40cm/s)	<0.4cm	0.4–1.0cm	>1cm
Pulmonary vein flow	Systolic dominant	Systolic blunting	Systolic flow reversal
Mitral inflow	A wave dominant	Variable	E wave dominant and >1.2m/s
Continuous wave Doppler	Soft, mild density, parabolic	Variable	Dense and triangular shape
Regurgitant fraction	<30%	30–50%	>50%
EROA (via PISA)	0–20mm^2	20–40mm^2	>40mm^2

Pitfalls in grading severity

Quantitative techniques are the most reliable and validated measurements but require time and operator experience.

Additional issues include:
- Eccentric jets—many quantitative measures are inaccurate
- Multiple jets—vena contracta and PISA inaccurate
- Atrial fibrillation—affects mitral valve and pulmonary vein flow
- Machine settings—adjustment in colour settings and Nyquist limit can radically alter appearance of the regurgitant jet.

Additional imaging

Transoesophageal echocardiography provides excellent anatomical and functional information and assists accurate quantitative assessment in almost all cases. Additional modalities may include:

- CMR (with late gadolinium)—assessment of LV function and areas of infarction (particularly if there is coexistent coronary artery disease).
- Radionuclide scan—accurate assessment of ejection fraction.
- 3D transoesophageal echocardiography—modelling of valve and annulus.

Dynamic imaging

The complex relationship between the valve leaflets, annulus, papillary muscles, and ventricular wall mean that the regurgitant volume can vary significantly with heart rate, loading conditions and ischaemia. Consequently, the true extent of MR is difficult to assess and quantify during a resting study. Ideally exercise echocardiography should be performed to quantify any change in MR with exercise and any secondary rise in pulmonary arterial systolic pressure.

Patients with a marked increase in MR during exercise are at increased risk of acute pulmonary oedema which may also be precipitated by tachycardia, ischaemia, increased afterload, and diastolic dysfunction.

Along with assessment of regurgitant severity, an objective measurement of ejection fraction and volume before and after exercise can be used to identify patients with sub-clinical LV dysfunction. Those without contractile reserve have poorer outcomes both before and after surgical intervention.

Invasive assessment

Cardiac catheterization and left ventriculography are rarely required for diagnosis and reserved for patients with a discrepancy between clinical symptoms/signs and echocardiographic findings. Right heart catheterization (with measurement of pulmonary arterial and wedge pressure) may be particularly useful in patients with dyspnoea and associated respiratory disease.

Surveillance

General measures

Education and counselling regarding potential symptoms and the need to seek medical attention should be provided to all patients. Asymptomatic patients should remain active and undertake symptom limited exercise. Regular blood pressure checks and appropriate treatment for other cardiovascular risk factors are appropriate.

Serial review

Asymptomatic patients should remain under regular review whose frequency is dependent on clinical and echocardiographic criteria:

Severity	Minimum review frequency
Mild to moderate	12 months clinical review—echocardiogram every 24 months
Severe	6 months clinical review—echocardiogram every 12 months
Borderline LV function	Consider review at 3–6 month intervals

Medical therapy

Surgery should be considered in all patients with associated with symptoms and/or LV impairment. Medical therapy should not be used to defer the need for surgery, but may be applicable for temporary symptomatic relief or palliation in those unsuitable for intervention:
- Diuretic therapy to reduce fluid overload
- ACE inhibitors, β blockers and aldosterone antagonists for LV dysfunction
- Warfarin (or an alternative vitamin K antagonist) for atrial fibrillation.

ACE inhibitors (or other vasodilators) are not recommended for patients with asymptomatic MR and normal LV function. They are, however, a logical choice in the patient with significant MR and associated hypertension.

Acute severe MR requires urgent surgical management—holding measures to stabilize the patient include:
- Opiates
- Intravenous diuretics
- Vasodilators, e.g. nitrates, sodium nitroprusside
- Inotropic agents, e.g. dobutamine
- Continuous positive airway pressure ventilation (CPAP)
- Intra-aortic balloon pump.

Indications for surgery

Acute mitral regurgitation

Acute severe MR associated with symptoms is an indication for immediate surgical intervention.

Chronic mitral regurgitation

Patients with severe chronic MR should be considered for surgery in the following situations:

Symptoms with no contraindication to surgery:
- Symptoms and ejection fraction (EF) >30% and LV end systolic diameter <55mm
- Severe LV dysfunction refractory to medical therapy and high likelihood of repair (EF <30% and/or LV end systolic diameter >55mm).

Asymptomatic with no contraindication to surgery:
- LV dysfunction—EF<60% and/or LV end systolic diameter >45mm
- Normal LV function with pulmonary hypertension (pulmonary artery systolic pressure >50mmHg)
- Normal LV function and atrial fibrillation.

Weighing the benefits of early surgery (before the development of LV dysfunction) against the small operative risks in individual patients is often difficult. Exact approaches will depend on local expertise and the likelihood of valve repair (see 🕮 p.276).

Mitral valve surgery in heart failure

Severe MR in patients with heart failure and poor LV function is a particular challenge when considering mitral valve repair or replacement. Correction of severe MR will unload the LV, but recovery of LV function may not always follow. Factors suggesting LV function recovery is likely include:
- Heart failure duration <5 years
- Preserved renal function
- LV end-diastolic diameter <80mm
- Reversible pulmonary hypertension
- Optimal medical therapy preoperatively (including use of cardiac resynchronisation therapy if appropriate).

The degree of LV contractile reserve can be assessed with dobutamine stress echocardiography, and CMR with gadolinium can be used to quantify the extent of myocardial fibrosis. If there is extensive myocardial scar and little or no demonstrable functional reserved then improvement (in both LV function and symptoms) following correction of MR is unlikely.

Mitral regurgitation and aortic regurgitation

The combination of MR and AR is occasionally identified in patients with pathologies affecting both valves e.g. IE, rheumatic valvular heart disease, ankylosing spondylitis or Marfan's syndrome.

Pathophysiology

AR increases LV pressure and elevates the LV to left atrial gradient thereby exacerbating the degree of MR. Both lesions lead to LV dilation but dominant AR may cause a degree of systemic hypertension and LV hypertrophy.

Echocardiographic assessment is usually straightforward and helps to clarify the dominant lesion. Exercise echocardiography may also be very useful to demonstrate dynamic changes.

Management

Management should be directed at the dominant lesion. If aortic valve replacement is required then concomitant mitral valve repair is the preferred option (if required) given the surgical challenge, morbidity and mortality associated with double valve replacement.

Management algorithm for severe mitral regurgitation

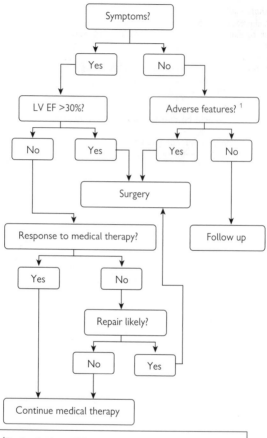

¹Ejection fraction ≤60%
Atrial fibrillation
LV systolic diameter >45mm
Peak RV systolic pressure >50mmHg at rest.

Tricuspid stenosis

Introduction

TS is a rare condition in the developed world—worldwide it is most commonly caused by rheumatic fever. It is usually an incidental finding and can be easily overlooked, especially if there is associated left sided valvular heart disease, e.g. MS. Rheumatic TS is usually accompanied by TR which makes assessment more complicated.

Aetiology

TS is a primary lesion of the valve leaflets and can be caused by:
- Rheumatic valvular heart disease—usually associated with TR (Fig. 8.1)
- IE—large obstructive vegetations
- Carcinoid—always associated with TR
- Congenital valve abnormalities
- Systemic lupus erythematosus
- Fabry's disease
- Whipple's disease
- Mechanical obstruction by thrombus
- Myxoma
- Pacemaker lead induced valve stenosis
- Trauma from long term indwelling central venous catheter
- Methysergide therapy.

Symptoms

Chronic TS may remain asymptomatic for many years as the right atrium and inferior vena cava dilate. After some time, these compensatory mechanisms may start to fail with development of symptoms, typically:
- Dyspnoea—initially on effort then at rest
- Prominent venous engorgement
- Peripheral oedema
- Abdominal distension
- Jaundice due to hepatic congestion.

Additional symptoms may relate to additional left sided disease, e.g. MS.

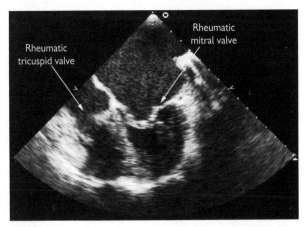

Fig. 8.1 Transoesophogeal echocardiogram—both the mitral and tricuspid valves are thickened secondary to rheumatic valvular heart disease.

Clinical signs

The jugular venous pulse is abnormal (giant a wave). A pre-systolic and mid-diastolic murmur is heard in inspiration and an opening snap may be identifiable (though frequently obscured by signs of mitral valve disease). Associated signs of TR are often present.

Other clinical signs relate to the development of RV failure and may include:
• Peripheral oedema
• Elevated venous pressure
• Jaundice.

Natural history

Severe TS can be tolerated for some time and may remain undiagnosed for years—the additional mitral valve disease often dominates and TS is often missed.

The association of severe TR may result in volume loading of the RV and makes management more complicated.

Initial investigations

Once TS is suspected definitive diagnosis is usually with echocardiography. The ECG and chest X-ray are usually non specific. Echocardiography is a very useful technique although RV function can be difficult to quantify (see 📖 p.68).

CMR is superior to echocardiography in the assessment of RV function and also allows assessment of the stenotic tricuspid valve. Radionuclide ventriculography can assess RV ejection fraction but provides no data on the valve itself.

Differential diagnosis

MS and TS are frequently mistaken for each other as the clinical signs are broadly similar.

Mechanical obstruction of right atrial outflow can mimic MS. Possible causes include:
• Intra-cardiac tumour
• Congenital membrane
• Right atrial thrombus
• Embolised tumour mass or thrombus
• Large vegetations obstructing tricuspid valve orifice.

Occasionally, the signs and symptoms of TS may be mistaken for constrictive pericarditis or restrictive cardiomyopathy; these should be readily identified at echocardiography.

Echocardiographic assessment

Full echocardiographic assessment should include the following:
• Severity of TS—colour flow and Doppler (Fig. 8.2)
• Valve morphology and mechanism
• Inferior vena cava and hepatic vein dilation, and response to inspiration
• Flow reversal in the hepatic veins (indicates severe TR)
• Measurement of RV systolic pressure from TR jet.

Given the high likelihood of additional MS careful assessment of the left heart is mandatory:
• Mitral valve anatomy and function
• LV systolic and diastolic dimensions
• LV ejection fraction.

Measurement of the pressure gradient and pressure half time are undertaken as described for MS (see 📖 p.162).

Transthoracic vs. transoesophageal echocardiography

Transoesophageal echocardiography is not as effective for assessment of the tricuspid valve in comparison with left sided lesions, but can provide additional anatomical information regarding leaflet morphology and function. Acquisition of accurate Doppler data for the tricuspid valve is difficult and a transthoracic study is often superior.

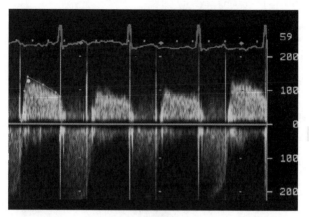

Fig. 8.2 Pulsed wave Doppler demonstrating flow through the tricuspid valve. The mean gradient measurement is 5mmHg, compatible with moderate to severe tricuspid stenosis.

Grading severity

Grading can be difficult and is determined by the haemodynamic significance of TS.

Severe TS is defined by:
• Mean pressure gradient ≥5mmHg
• Pressure half-time ≥190ms.

Pitfalls in grading severity

The severity of TS may be underestimated in:
• Significant associated TR
• Off axis Doppler measurements—particularly with transoesophageal echocardiography.

Invasive assessment

Cardiac catheterization is seldom undertaken solely for the diagnosis of TS. Nevertheless, the pressure gradient across the tricuspid valve can be measured if necessary. Since the right heart pressures are low, simultaneous recording of right atrial and RV pressure using two catheters (averaged over at least 10 cardiac cycles) is mandatory to obtain an accurate recording.

Many patients with MS require left and right heart catheterization prior to intervention, at which time the tricuspid valve can also be assessed. Since TS is frequently missed at echocardiography, documentation of an abnormal tricuspid pressure gradient may influence treatment and surgical strategy.

Medical therapy

General measures

Medical therapy is directed at relief of symptoms, primarily by reducing fluid overload with the use of loop diuretics. Spironolactone may also help, especially to prevent hypokalaemia.

Additional treatment may be required for the control of atrial fibrillation.

Surveillance

General measures

Patient education with regard to specific symptoms is useful:
• Worsening dyspnoea or reduced exercise tolerance
• Increasing pitting oedema
• Abdominal swelling and bloating
• Anorexia and jaundice.

The development of these new symptoms should prompt re-evaluation of the TS.

Serial review

The need for repeat clinical and echocardiographic assessment is dependent on the severity of symptoms and the presence of additional mitral valve disease.

Indications for surgery

Surgery is rarely undertaken for isolated severe TS and reserved for those with severe symptoms refractory to medical therapy. A lower threshold is adopted if surgery is being undertaken for associated mitral valve disease.

Surgical therapy

Valve repair is preferable to replacement where feasible. Surgical commissurotomy may be performed in selected cases but carries a risk of inducing TR.

Tricuspid valve replacement is usually required and should employ the largest possible prosthesis. As right heart pressures and flow are low the risk of thrombosis of a prosthetic valve is at least equal to that for mitral prostheses, if not higher. A bioprosthetic valve may be preferred to reduce this risk and has good long term outcomes in many patients.

Percutaneous tricuspid valvuloplasty is technically feasible but rarely performed (see 📖 p.318).

TS in patients needing CABG

There is usually no indication for tricuspid valve intervention in patients undergoing primary CABG. If TS is significant and likely to cause residual symptoms then concomitant valve surgery can be considered (especially if there is associated mitral valve disease).

Tricuspid regurgitation

Introduction

A degree of TR is found in the majority of patients at echocardiography and is clinically insignificant. It is important however to detect more severe TR as it can lead to severe symptoms and poor prognosis.

TR may be a consequence of damage to the tricuspid valve leaflets but is more commonly secondary to RV dilation and dysfunction. The importance of TR in determining the outcome of patients with aortic and mitral valve disease undergoing surgery has only recently been fully appreciated.

Epidemiology

Asymptomatic, clinically undetectable TR is found in two thirds of adults undergoing echocardiography. More significant TR is uncommon, and found in only 10–15% of patients over 65 years of age. Severe TR due to a primary valve abnormality is very rare.

Aetiology

TR is usually secondary to dilation of the RV and tricuspid annulus, so called 'functional' TR. A primary lesion of the valve leaflets is less likely.

Primary valve lesion

Lesions directly affecting the tricuspid valve are rare. Congenital abnormalities of the valve leaflets may be found in young patients and infective endocarditis (IE) affecting the tricuspid valve in intravenous drug users is increasingly frequent.

Valvular abnormalities

- Ebstein's anomaly
- Cleft valve (associated with other malformations)
- IE (Fig. 9.1)
- Rheumatic valvular heart disease
- Carcinoid syndrome (Fig. 9.2)
- Prolapse—sometimes associated with mitral valve prolapse
- Rheumatoid arthritis
- Systemic lupus erythematosus
- Radiation damage
- Marfan's syndrome
- Dopamine agonists e.g. pergolide, cabergoline, fenfluramine.

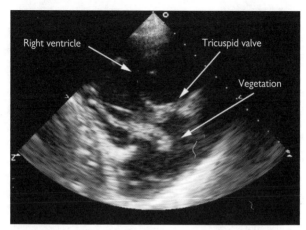

Fig. 9.1 Right ventricular view from a parasternal position. A large vegetation (arrowed) is seen attached to the posterior tricuspid valve leaflet and prolapsing into the right atrium.

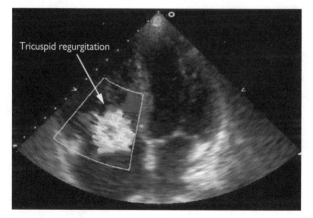

Fig. 9.2 A very broad jet of TR on colour flow Doppler—the tricuspid leaflets are fixed in an open position due to carcinoid disease. See also **Plate 15.**

Secondary tricuspid regurgitation

Any pathology causing dilation of the RV can lead to TR. Causes can be divided as follows:

Pressure loaded RV
- LV failure
- Left sided valvular heart disease—usually MR or MS
- Chronic thromboembolic disease (Fig. 9.3)
- PS
- Pulmonary artery stenosis
- Intrinsic respiratory disease (*cor pulmonale*)
- Primary (idiopathic) pulmonary hypertension

Volume overloaded RV
- RV infarction
- Shunt e.g. atrial septal defect
- RV cardiomyopathy e.g. arrhythmogenic RV dysplasia

Iatrogenic
- Pacemaker lead induced TR
- Endocardial biopsy

Other causes
- Atrial fibrillation—can cause right atrial dilation
- Hyperthyroidism

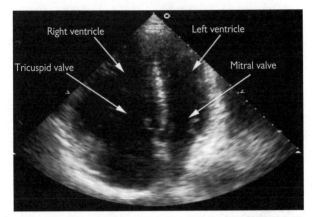

Fig. 9.3 A severely dilated RV (much larger than the LV) with clear dilation of the tricuspid valve annulus secondary to pulmonary hypertension following recurrent pulmonary emboli.

Symptoms

Chronic TR may remain asymptomatic for many years as the RV copes with increased stroke volume. Compensatory mechanisms eventually fail and symptoms develop, typically:
- Dyspnoea—initially on effort then at rest
- Prominent venous engorgement
- Peripheral oedema
- Abdominal distension
- Jaundice due to hepatic congestion
- Awareness of increased pulsation in neck and head.

Clinical signs

The increased stroke volume in TR is usually clinically silent. Abnormal physical findings may include:
- Elevated venous pressure with marked 'CV' waves—vigorous systolic waves which can be mistaken for arterial pulsation
- Increased venous distension on inspiration
- Pansystolic murmur at left sternal edge (Rivero–Carvallo's sign)
- RV heave
- RV third heart sound
- Pulsatile liver
- Systolic thrill over jugular vein.

Other clinical signs relate to the development of ventricular failure and include:
- Peripheral oedema
- Jaundice
- Hypotension due to reduced LV filling.

Rare clinical signs which have been described are:
- Pulsatile varicosities
- Pulsation of the orbits.

Examination should also focus on the underlying aetiology of TR with particular focus on the aortic and mitral valves, LV function and pulmonary disease.

Natural history

TR typically follows a slow course with very gradual progression. There is, however, marked inter-individual variation since TR is most frequently due to additional pathology of the left heart or pulmonary circulation, the natural history of these conditions may dominate.

Severe TR is associated with adverse outcomes—one year survival is 64% compared with 92% in patients with only mild TR (even after adjustment for LV dysfunction or pulmonary hypertension).

TR due to RV dilation or left sided lesions may persist after treatment of the underlying condition—predictors include residual pulmonary hypertension, annular dilation and poor RV function.

Initial investigations

Definitive diagnosis is usually confirmed with echocardiography. The ECG and chest X-ray are usually non specific but may reveal the underlying aetiology.

ECG

There are no specific ECG changes in TR—abnormalities usually result from effects on the RV or the underlying aetiology (e.g. RV infarction) and may include:

- Inferior or posterior ischaemia/infarction
- Right pre-cordial lead ST or T wave changes
- RV hypertrophy and right axis deviation
- Atrial fibrillation.

Chest X-ray

RV enlargement is the typical finding. There may be changes relating to the underlying cardiac or pulmonary aetiology:

- LV enlargement
- Right atrial enlargement
- Pleural effusions
- Liver enlargement causing an elevated diaphragm
- Prominent pulmonary arteries.

Differential diagnosis

The murmur of TR may be mistaken for:

- Ventricular septal defect—also pan-systolic and left sternal edge
- MR—usually radiates to the axilla.

The abnormal jugular venous pressure must be distinguished from:

- TS—prominent a wave
- Congestive cardiac failure—no v wave
- Complete heart block—cannon waves
- Superior vena cava obstruction—non pulsatile
- Constrictive pericarditis—venous pressure rises markedly on inspiration.

Echocardiographic assessment

The tricuspid valve is challenging to fully assess with echocardiography due to its anterior location and relation to the sternum. There is also considerable variation in the size of the three leaflets—the anterior leaflet is in a consistent position but the posterior and septal leaflets can vary in their size and point of insertion.

Furthermore, grading the severity of TR is difficult due to dependence on loading conditions. Appropriate detailed clinical assessment should always be integrated with the results of echocardiography.

The tricuspid valve should be visualized as fully as possible to document:
• Leaflet size and location
• Leaflet thickness and mobility
• Location of TR
• Degree of TR
• Size of annulus
• Size of right atrium and RV
• RV function
• Estimation of RV systolic pressure.

Given that aetiology is usually secondary to additional cardiac or pulmonary pathology, the following should also be carefully assessed:
• LV systolic and diastolic dimensions
• LV ejection fraction
• Ventricular septal motion
• Aortic and mitral valve function
• Inferior vena cava and hepatic vein dilation—response to inspiration
• Flow reversal in the hepatic veins—indicates severe TR
• Inter-atrial septal motion—may suggest high right atrial pressure
• Pulmonary valve and pulmonary artery morphology.

Leaflet size and location

Echocardiographic assessment can identify the pathology causing the TR. An abnormal valve, dilated annulus, IE with vegetations or cusp destruction can all be demonstrated (Fig. 9.4).

The degree of apical offset of the annular plane relative to the mitral valve should be scrutinized to ensure that Ebstein's anomaly is not overlooked. Three-dimensional echocardiography provides improved anatomical information and facilitates identification of the valve leaflets.

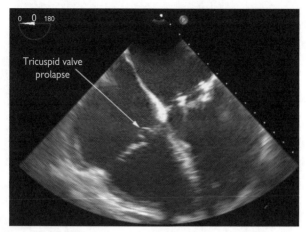

Fig. 9.4 Transoesophogeal echocardiogram demonstrating severe tricuspid regurgitation due to prolapse of the septal leaflet (arrowed).

Degree of regurgitation

Colour flow Doppler is a highly sensitive method for the detection and visualization of TR. In conjunction with continuous wave Doppler, this provides accurate quantification of the severity of regurgitation.

Eccentric jets which entrain along the atrial wall are more challenging to quantify.

Right ventricular size and function

The size and shape of the RV should be assessed with measurement of the ventricular cavity dimensions in end-diastole (Fig. 9.5). Right ventricular systolic function can be estimated using TAPSE (see 📖 p.68). If this measurement is not possible, then radionuclide ventriculography or CMR imaging may be used to measure RV ejection fraction.

Inferior vena cava and hepatic vein flow

The size of the inferior vena cava and its response to inspiration can be used to estimate right atrial pressure.

Right atrial pressure (mmHg)	0–5	5–10	10–15	15–20	>20
Inferior vena cava size (cm)	<1.5	1.5–2.5	1.5–2.5	>2.5	>2.5
Respiratory variation	Collapse	↓<50%	↓<50%	↓<50%	No change

Pulsed wave Doppler interrogation of flow in the hepatic veins is used to identify severe TR. Similar to flow reversal in the pulmonary veins associated with MR, flow reversal in the hepatic veins during systole suggests severe TR. Atrial fibrillation reduces the accuracy of this technique.

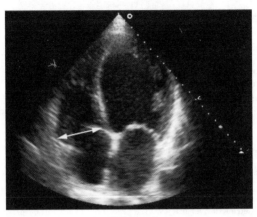

Fig. 9.5 The basal dimension of the RV (arrowed).

Transthoracic vs. transoesophageal echocardiography

Imaging the tricuspid valve with transoesophageal echocardiography is often more difficult as the thin leaflets are further from the probe and may be obscured by shadowing from the aortic and mitral valves.

Imaging from the low oesophagus and transgastric position can assist visualisation of the valve leaflets but obtaining accurate alignment with any regurgitant jet can be hard.

Transoesophageal echocardiography is very useful in patients with suspected tricuspid valve IE or those with pacing or defibrillator electrodes in place —the relationship to the valve leaflets and chordal apparatus may be relevant to the mechanism of regurgitation.

Grading severity

The severity of TR can be graded as:
- Trace (physiological)
- Mild
- Moderate
- Severe.

Severity of TR is very dependent on loading conditions and these must be taken into account—TR may appear more severe before the initiation of diuretic therapy.

Severe TR is defined on echocardiography as:
- Systolic flow reversal in hepatic veins
- Vena contracta width >7mm (Fig. 9.6)
- PISA radius ≥9mm (with Nyquist limit set at 40cm/s).

Other associated findings include:
- Triangular shaped Doppler—dense signal with early peak (Fig. 9.7)
- Dilated inferior vena cava with severely reduced inspiratory variation
- Trans-tricuspid peak E wave >1m/s
- RV and right atrial dilation suggesting volume overload.

Pitfalls in grading severity

The severity of TR can be underestimated in:
- RV failure
- Eccentric jets
- Poor acoustic windows
- Hypovolaemia.

Avoiding assessment error
- Use venous injection of agitated saline to improve Doppler signal
- Combine imaging assessment with clinical signs
- Consider alternative imaging strategies.

CMR imaging may be required to provide accurate assessment of RV anatomy, function and myocardial appearances (scar formation and fatty replacement).

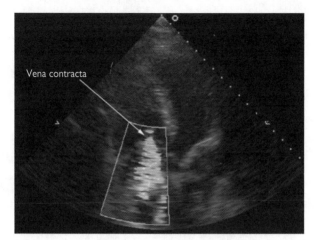

Fig. 9.6 Transthoracic echocardiogram with colour flow mapping of TR demonstrating the vena contracta. See also **Plate 16.**

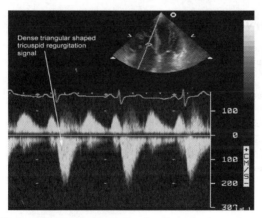

Fig. 9.7 Severe TR on continuous wave Doppler—the signal is dense and triangular in shape with a peak in early systole.

Invasive assessment

Right heart catheterization is seldom required to confirm the diagnosis of TR but may be undertaken to clarify the aetiology and provide accurate measurement of RV, pulmonary arterial and left atrial pressures.

If surgery to treat the underlying cause (e.g. MR) is planned then left and right heart catheterization (including coronary angiography) should be performed (see 📖 p.82).

Medical therapy

General measures

Management of TR is directed at:
• Treatment of underlying aetiology
• Reducing pulmonary hypertension
• Reducing venous pressure.

Symptoms can be improved with loop diuretics to reduce RV volume overload and hepatic congestion. Spironolactone may also help to prevent hypokalaemia. If pulmonary hypertension is the prime aetiology then pulmonary vasodilators (sildenafil or bosentan) may be used in appropriate cases.

Surveillance

General measures

Patient education with regard to specific symptoms is useful:
• Worsening dyspnoea and reduced exercise tolerance
• Increasing peripheral oedema
• Abdominal swelling and bloating
• Anorexia and jaundice.

Development of these symptoms should prompt re-evaluation of the TR.

Serial review

The frequency of assessment is largely dictated by the underlying aetiology, RV function, and presence of symptoms. Asymptomatic moderate TR with a good RV can remain asymptomatic and stable for many years.

Indications for surgery

Primary tricuspid regurgitation

If a primary problem with the tricuspid valve causes TR then surgical correction should be considered in the following scenarios:

- Severe symptomatic TR without severe RV impairment
- Severe asymptomatic TR with progressive dilation or impairment of RV function.

Severe RV dysfunction is a significant contributor to poor outcome following tricuspid valve surgery. Irreversible RV remodelling is unlikely to improve with valve surgery.

Re-do surgery for tricuspid regurgitation

Severe TR may develop late after initial surgery on the aortic or mitral valve and is associated with poor prognosis. Re-do sternotomy to allow tricuspid annuloplasty carries a significant risk (approximately 10–20% mortality) and should only be contemplated in patients with:

- Symptomatic severe TR
- Normal RV function
- No residual aortic or mitral valve disease
- Good LV function
- Normal pulmonary arterial pressure.

Secondary tricuspid regurgitation

Since TR is usually secondary to other cardiac or pulmonary pathology, a common clinical scenario is the patient requiring cardiac surgery for another reason (e.g. correction of MR) who may also require tricuspid valve repair or replacement. The decision to intervene on the tricuspid valve is based on the following considerations:

- TR is not guaranteed to resolve when mitral or aortic valve pathology is corrected, and may in fact progress to severe long after surgery
- As many as 50% of patients with MR needing surgery will have significant tricuspid annular dilation, even in the absence of significant TR
- Late TR is associated with poor prognosis in patients undergoing aortic or mitral valve surgery
- Tricuspid annuloplasty is relatively low risk when performed at the time of mitral or aortic valve surgery and can be performed quickly once the aortic cross clamp is removed
- The tricuspid valve tolerates imperfect repair—total competence is not essential
- Re-do surgery to correct severe TR is frequently a high-risk procedure.

Mild degrees of TR do not require surgical treatment.

Indications for tricuspid annuloplasty

Surgical intervention (preferably annuloplasty) should be undertaken in patients undergoing mitral or aortic valve surgery with:

• Severe TR
• Moderate TR and annular diameter >40mm (or >21mm/body surface area).

The risk of a patient developing progressive TR after mitral or aortic valve surgery should also be considered—in some cases early repair may be justified. Risk factors associated with progressive TR include:

• Increasing age
• Female gender
• Rheumatic valvular heart disease
• Atrial fibrillation
• Elevated pulmonary arterial pressure.

Surgical therapy

The choice of operative procedure (repair versus replacement) depends on the pathology of regurgitation and the anatomy of the tricuspid annulus. Detailed assessment is required. In general tricuspid repair is preferred due to the high thrombo-embolic potential of a prosthetic tricuspid valve.

Tricuspid valve repair

Repair techniques using an annuloplasty ring to reduce annular size are the mainstay of treatment for secondary TR. An experienced operator and team are essential. Careful preoperative assessment with transoesophageal echocardiography is required to assess the lesion and suitability for repair.

Long term results of tricuspid annuloplasty are reasonable with only 10% of patients having significant residual TR at 5 years. However, operative mortality can be high (>20%) depending on the underlying aetiology, and long term follow up suggests only a 50% 10 year survival.

For primary TR there may be a role for valve sparing surgery and neochordal implantation in addition to insertion of an annuloplasty ring. There are very few expert surgeons offering this type of reconstructive surgery. Long term follow up data are lacking due to the small numbers of patients treated.

Tricuspid valve replacement

If repair is not possible, then valve replacement is an option. However, it may be wiser to avoid valve replacement altogether, especially if correction of an associated left sided valve lesion is expected to reduce secondary TR. If the tricuspid valve is diseased and cannot be repaired, then a large bioprosthesis is advocated to reduce the risk of prosthetic valve thrombosis.

If there is evidence of pre-existing conduction tissue disease then permanent epicardial pacing leads should be implanted in anticipation of being unable to perform transvenous pacing.

Survival following tricuspid valve replacement is poor—early studies demonstrated a 5 year survival rate of only 45%.

Tricuspid regurgitation in patients needing CABG

There is no indication for tricuspid valve intervention in patients undergoing primary CABG, unless the degree of TR is thought to be sufficiently severe to curtail the benefits of the intended coronary artery surgery.

Pulmonary stenosis

Introduction

PS is a relatively rare condition and almost always congenital in origin. Associations with sub- or supra-valvar stenosis are common, and more complex congenital lesions such as Fallot's tetralogy should be considered (Fig. 10.1). PS is usually an incidental finding in the adult population which can be easily overlooked, especially if there is left-sided valvular heart disease.

Epidemiology

PS is found in up to 10% of congenital heart disease patients, with a slight preponderance in females. Most cases present in childhood with a benign clinical course.

Aetiology

True PS is a primary lesion of the valve leaflets.
- Congenital valve abnormalities—cusp numbers can vary.
- Carcinoid—always associated with PR (predominant feature).
- Rheumatic valvular heart disease—usually associated with PR.
- Congenital rubella.
- Noonan's syndrome—short stature and webbed neck.
- Watson's syndrome—cafe-au-lait spots and cognitive impairment.
- William's syndrome—elfin face, wide mouth, small chin.
- Alagille syndrome—broad forehead, pointed chin, long nose.
- IE—large vegetations.
- Extrinsic compression—tumour.
- Complex lesions—e.g. Fallot's, univentricular heart, double outlet RV.
- Pseudovalvar stenosis (sub- or supra-valvar)—membranes, extrinsic compression, pulmonary artery stenosis.

In the typical case of congenital PS, the valve leaflets are thickened and fused with doming in systole. Calcification of the leaflets is rare.

Noonan's syndrome is associated with valve dysplasia and hypoplasia of the annulus and proximal pulmonary artery—surgery in early childhood is invariably required.

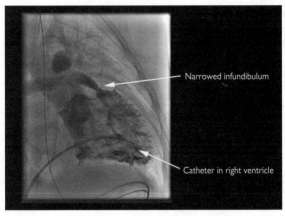

Fig. 10.1 Narrow infundibulum and restricted pulmonary valve in a patient with Fallot's tetralogy.

Symptoms

Chronic PS may remain asymptomatic for many years as the RV hypertrophies and the right atrium dilates. After some time these compensatory mechanisms fail with the development of symptoms:
- Dyspnoea
- Fatigue
- Exertional syncope.

Signs in late stage disease include:
- Prominent venous engorgement
- Peripheral oedema
- Abdominal distension
- Hepatic congestion.

Clinical signs

The signs may be subtle—the jugular venous pulse is usually normal but may demonstrate a prominent a wave. An ejection systolic murmur is heard in the pulmonary area. The second heart sound (P2) may be quiet but also split due to delayed pulmonary valve closure. A parasternal heave may be detected if there is significant RV hypertrophy, and a RV fourth heart sound may develop in RV failure.

Other clinical signs relate to the development of ventricular failure and include:
- Peripheral oedema
- Elevated venous pressure
- Jaundice
- Cyanosis—if elevated right sided pressures promote right to left shunting through an atrial septal defect or patent foramen ovale.

Natural history

Severe PS can be tolerated for some time and remain undiagnosed for years. Isolated PS usually has a benign prognosis. Sudden cardiac death is rare.

Initial investigations

The ECG may reveal changes of right atrial and RV hypertrophy/dilation with P pulmonale, and right axis deviation.

The chest X-ray may demonstrate dilated pulmonary arteries (post-stenotic dilation) with oligaemic lung fields if there is severe obstruction. Rarely there may be vascular fullness at the left base due to preferential flow of the stenotic jet into the left pulmonary artery (Chen's sign).

Once PS is suspected, the definitive diagnosis is confirmed with echocardiography. The pulmonary valve may be hard to demonstrate with transthoracic imaging but can usually be seen with a combination of parasternal short axis and modified subcostal views. Continuous wave Doppler assessment through the pulmonary valve to determine the peak and mean pressure drop is required to confirm valvular stenosis and assess its severity. As in AS, the valve area can be estimated using the continuity equation (see ☐ p.62).

Care must be taken when quantifying pulmonary artery systolic pressure using the TR signal as the standard simplified Bernoulli equation is only valid in the absence of PS—the modified Bernoulli's equation should be used.

Pressure drop = 4 × (peak TR velocity^2 − peak PS velocity^2)

CMR imaging is more accurate for assessment of RV volume and function, and can provide accurate imaging of the right ventricular outflow tract, including planimetry of valve area and estimation of peak velocity across the valve (Fig. 10.2).

Differential diagnosis

It is more usual to miss PS than mistake it for an alternative diagnosis. However, the murmur may be misinterpreted as AS or a ventricular septal defect.

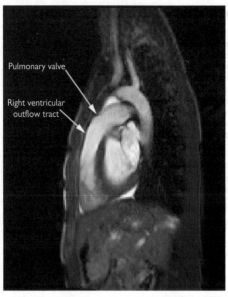

Fig. 10.2 CMR image of the right ventricular outflow tract and pulmonary valve (arrowed).

Echocardiographic assessment

A full echocardiographic assessment should include the following:
- RV systolic and diastolic dimensions
- RV ejection fraction
- RV function
- Severity of PS—colour flow and Doppler
- Inferior vena cava and hepatic vein dilation
- Inferior vena cava response to inspiration (Fig. 10.3)
- Valve morphology and mechanism of PS
- Measurement of RV systolic pressure from TR jet (modified Bernoulli)
- Hepatic vein Doppler (Fig. 10.3)
- Other valve lesions.

Severity assessment—Doppler

Continuous wave Doppler provides accurate quantification of the severity of stenosis (Fig. 10.4).

Valve morphology

Assessment with transthoracic and transoesophageal echocardiography can facilitate identification of the pathological process underlying PS. An abnormal valve, extrinsic compression, IE with vegetations, or cusp destruction can all be identified (Fig. 10.5).

Associated abnormalities

Identification of additional valvular heart disease and quantification of LV and RV function (including assessment of pulmonary arterial pressure) are required to fully assess a patient with PS.

Transthoracic vs. transoesophageal echocardiography

The pulmonary valve is difficult to image with either modality—a transoesophageal study is rarely required in the routine assessment of PS. Conversely, if IE of the pulmonary valve is suspected, then a transoesophageal echocardiography is essential.

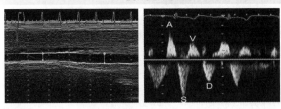

Fig. 10.3 Left hand panel shows M-mode interrogation of the inferior vena cava during inspiration—minimum and maximum diameters are marked. The right hand panel is an example of pulsed wave Doppler flow in the hepatic veins—the normal phases of venous flow are labelled.

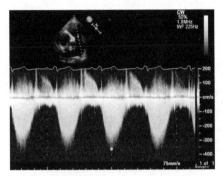

Fig. 10.4 Continuous wave Doppler in severe PS—the peak velocity is close to 4m/s (peak gradient 50mmHg).

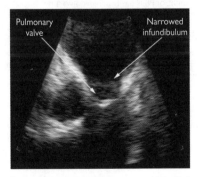

Fig. 10.5 Transthoracic image demonstrating a narrowed infundibulum and dysplastic pulmonary valve with fused leaflets.

Grading severity

PS is defined on continuous wave Doppler echocardiography as follows:

	Mild	Moderate	Severe
Peak gradient (mmHg)	10 – 20	25 – 40	>40
Valve area (cm^2)	> 1.0	0.5 – 1.0	< 0.5

Severe PS is suggested on echocardiography by:
• Severe RV hypertrophy; at least 5mm wall thickness
• Right atrial dilation
• RV dilation suggests a failing ventricle.

Pitfalls in grading severity

The severity of PS can be misjudged in:
• The presence of dilation of the pulmonary artery distal to the valve
• The presence of significant PR
• Significant pulmonary hypertension
• Off axis assessment during Doppler measurement—not uncommon in older subjects.

Avoiding assessment error

• Combine imaging assessment with clinical signs and ECG findings
• Consider alternative imaging strategies, e.g., CMR, cardiac catheterization.

Invasive assessment

Invasive assessment of PS is easily achieved via a right heart catheter study but rarely required unless intervention is planned or multiple levels of stenosis are suspected. Direct measurement of right atrial, RV, and pulmonary arterial pressure may also be of use to guide further therapy.

Note that Doppler-derived gradients tend to be greater than those measured invasively. Thresholds for intervention in PS have historically been based on invasive data.

Medical therapy

General measures
Treatment is aimed at controlling symptoms and reducing fluid overload. Loop diuretics have a role in reducing RV pressure, volume overload, and hepatic congestion. Spironolactone may also help, especially to prevent hypokalaemia. Medical therapy for pulmonary hypertension is not usually required.

Surveillance

General measures
Patient education with regard to specific symptoms is useful:
- Worsening dyspnoea
- Reduced exercise tolerance
- Syncope
- Pitting oedema
- Abdominal swelling and bloating
- Anorexia and jaundice.

The development of these symptoms should prompt re-evaluation of the PS.

Serial review
Severe PS can be well tolerated for many years. The frequency of serial review is determined by the underlying cause. Clinical examination, ECG, and transthoracic echocardiography are the mainstay of follow up.

Surgical therapy

Intervention to relieve PS is ideally performed with balloon valvuloplasty (see 📖 p.316).

Surgery to relieve obstruction or replace the pulmonary valve (usually with a homograft) is indicated in:
• Failed balloon valvuloplasty with severe post procedural PR.
• Severe PS and complex congenital lesion.
• Pulmonary valve hypoplasia (Noonan's syndrome).

The choice of operation and technique (repair or replacement) depends on the pathology of the lesion and anatomy of the pulmonary annulus. Detailed assessment is required.

Pulmonary valve repair

Repair techniques for PS are limited due to the lack of available adjacent tissue—the pulmonary valve is usually too diseased to repair. If feasible, careful pre-operative assessment with transoesophageal echocardiography is required to assess the lesion classification and suitability for repair. Long term follow up data are lacking due to the small numbers of patients undergoing this type of surgery.

Pulmonary valve replacement

If the pulmonary valve is diseased but cannot be repaired and needs to be replaced, then either a homograft or bioprosthesis is preferred to a mechanical valve to reduce the risk of prosthetic valve thrombosis and need for lifelong anticoagulation. Bioprosthetic implants usually have a satisfactory lifespan in the pulmonary position.

Pulmonary regurgitation

Epidemiology

A trace of PR is detected in many subjects but clinically significant PR is rare. PR is usually secondary to previous intervention on the valve or outflow tract in the context of underlying congenital heart disease. IE of the pulmonary valve is extremely rare but can lead to significant PR.

Aetiology

Moderate PR in adults is commonly due to pulmonary hypertension, most cases of which relate to left sided ventricular or valvular disease.

Severe PR in adults can be due to:
• Previous intervention
  • Balloon valvuloplasty for PS
  • Pulmonary valve replacement (Fig. 11.1)
  • Repair of congenital heart disease e.g. Fallot's tetralogy
• Idiopathic dilation of the pulmonary artery
• IE
• Connective tissue disorders
• Carcinoid disease—but always associated with tricuspid valve disease.

Fallot's repair

Repair of Fallot's tetralogy involves closure of the ventricular septal defect, debulking of the infundibular muscle bundles and, often, enlargement of the RV outflow tract using a trans-annular patch to ensure no residual obstruction.

This combined procedure invariably leads to PR. More advanced techniques sparing the pulmonary valve or using a valved conduit have been developed but long term results are poor.

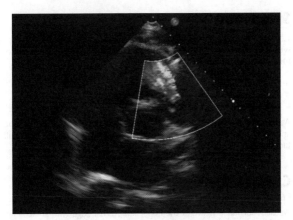

Fig. 11.1 Pulmonary regurgitation demonstrated on echocardiography in a patient with previous pulmonary valve replacement with a homograft. See also **Plate 17.**

Symptoms

Chronic PR may remain asymptomatic for many years as the RV copes well with the increased stroke volume. Eventually these compensatory mechanisms fail and symptoms develop:
• Dyspnoea—initially on effort, then at rest
• Peripheral oedema
• Abdominal distension
• Jaundice due to hepatic congestion.

Atrial arrhythmias, such as atrial fibrillation and atrial flutter, are common and ventricular scarring following surgery can act as a focus for ventricular tachycardia.

Clinical signs

The increased stroke volume in PR may be clinically silent. If present, a systolic murmur is heard at the upper left sternal edge with an accompanying early diastolic murmur at the lower left sternal edge.

Other clinical signs relate to the development of ventricular failure and include:
• Peripheral oedema
• Elevated venous pressure
• Jaundice.

The principal complication is the development of progressive RV dilation, impairment of systolic function, and heart failure. Marked RV dilation and impairment has a negative impact on LV filling with resultant LV failure.

Natural history

Severe PR can be tolerated for many years. However, the presence of RV dilation with poor systolic function predicts an increased incidence of ventricular arrhythmias and sudden cardiac death.

Initial investigations

The clinical diagnosis of PR is usually confirmed with echocardiography. The ECG typically shows right bundle branch block due to RV dilation or dysfunction.

Contrast angiography of the RV outflow tract and pulmonary arteries is performed to assess valve anatomy and function prior to intervention (Fig. 11.2).

CMR imaging can provide more accurate data on RV volume, and function, along with the anatomy of the RV outflow tract and pulmonary trunk.

Differential diagnosis

The diastolic murmur at the lower left sternal edge could be mimicked by AR, although the systolic flow murmur should be heard in the upper right parasternal area with the added sign of a collapsing carotid pulse.

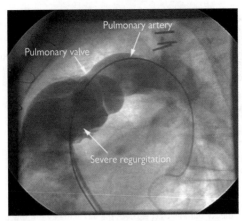

Fig. 11.2 Pulmonary angiography performed via right heart catheterization—note dense contrast below the pulmonary valve.

Echocardiographic assessment

Severity assessment—colour flow and Doppler

Colour flow Doppler is a highly sensitive method for the detection of PR (Fig.11.3). In conjunction with continuous wave Doppler, quantification of the severity of regurgitation is possible (Fig. 11.4).

Grading severity

The severity of PR can be graded as:
- Mild (physiological)
- Moderate
- Severe.

Severe PR is defined on echocardiography as:
- Colour jet fills the RV outflow tract
- Regurgitant fraction >60%
- Continuous wave Doppler regurgitant flow is steep and dense
- PISA radius ≥9mm (with Nyquist limit set at 40cm/s)
- VTI in the RV outflow tract exceeds the VTI in the LV outflow tract.

Valve morphology

Assessment with transthoracic or transoesophageal echocardiography facilitates identification of the pathology underlying PR. An abnormal valve, dilated annulus, IE with vegetations, or cusp destruction can all be identified.

Associated abnormalities

Identification of additional valvular heart disease and quantification of LV and RV function (including assessment of pulmonary arterial pressure) is required to fully assess a patient with PR.

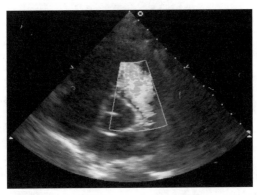

Fig.11.3 Colour flow Doppler demonstrating a broad jet of pulmonary regurgitation. See also **Plate 18.**

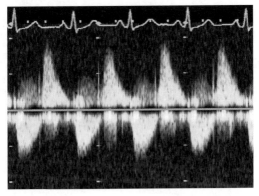

Fig. 11.4 Continuous wave Doppler demonstrating a broad jet of severe pulmonary regurgitation with rapid deceleration.

Medical therapy

General measures

Treatment is aimed at the relief of symptoms and control of fluid overload. Loop diuretics have a role in reducing RV volume overload and hepatic congestion. Spironolactone may also help, especially to prevent hypokalaemia. Pulmonary vasodilators such as bosentan and sildenafil may help if there is associated pulmonary hypertension—specialist input is required before their use.

LV dysfunction with secondary pulmonary hypertension will exacerbate PR—treatment with ACE inhibitors and diuretics is helpful.

Surveillance

General measures

Patient education with regard to specific symptoms is useful:
- Worsening dyspnoea/exercise tolerance
- Increasing pitting oedema
- Abdominal swelling and bloating
- Anorexia and jaundice.

The development of these symptoms should prompt re-evaluation of the PR and RV function.

Serial review

Severe PR can be tolerated for many years and the frequency of serial review should be determined by the underlying cause. Clinical examination, ECG and transthoracic echocardiography are the mainstay of follow up. The presence of worsening RV dilation and systolic dysfunction should prompt careful review.

Indications for surgery

Surgical intervention for isolated PR is usually only required in patients who have undergone prior surgery to the outflow tract e.g. Fallot's repair.

Surgical intervention should be considered in patients with:
- Symptoms despite medical therapy
- Moderate or severe RV dilation (Fig. 11.5)
- Clinically significant arrhythmia
- Significant RV dysfunction.

RV volumes assessed with CMR can guide the timing of intervention—end diastolic volumes >170ml/m2 or end systolic volumes > 85ml/m2 are associated with persistent RV enlargement following surgery.

Implantation of a balloon expandable stent containing a bovine venous valve across the pulmonary valve is a newly developed procedure which may prevent the need for high risk re-do surgery in many patients (See 📖 p.318).

Surgical therapy

The choice of procedure (repair or replacement) depends on the pathology of PR and the anatomy of the pulmonary annulus. Detailed assessment is required.

Pulmonary valve repair

Careful pre-operative assessment with CMR and transoesophageal echocardiography is required to assess the lesion and its suitability for repair.

Long term results of valve repair suggest that redo surgery, either for valvular stenosis of regurgitation is likely in at least 50% of subjects.

Pulmonary valve replacement

If the pulmonary valve is diseased but cannot be repaired and needs to be replaced then a homograft or bioprosthesis is usually recommended to reduce the risk of prosthetic valve thrombosis. Long term failure may well require further intervention.

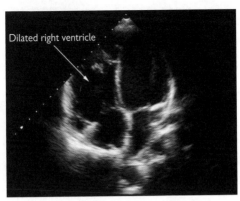

Fig. 11.5 Apical 4-chamber view demonstrating a significantly dilated RV secondary to volume loading.

Surgery and prosthetic valves

Introduction

A prosthetic valve of any form is an imperfect substitute for a native valve. Careful consideration of the long term consequences of valve surgery is therefore required and the optimum solution for each patient chosen.

Implications of prosthetic valves include:
• Abnormal flow haemodynamics
• Smaller orifice area compared to a native valve
• Limited durability
• Increased risk of thromboembolism
• Increased risk of IE
• Increased risk of further cardiac surgery.

A durable valve repair is therefore preferable to valve replacement wherever possible.

Preoperative assessment

As well as the standard assessment of a patient with valvular heart disease (See 📖 p.42), additional investigations may be required to assist surgical planning and risk assessment. These may include:
• Carotid Doppler—significant carotid disease?
• Pulmonary function tests—underlying impairment?
• Dental review—significant dental disease should be treated.

The impact of a thoracotomy on respiratory function is significant—vital capacity falls by 25% and takes 4–6 weeks to return to baseline.

Major complications of cardiac surgery should be considered and anticipated to allow pre-operative assessment—e.g. investigation and treatment of renal impairment discovered during routine preoperative screening.

Potential complications of cardiac surgery include:
• Myocardial ischaemia
• Respiratory impairment
• Acute renal failure
• Gastritis
• Mesenteric ischaemia
• Stroke
• Cognitive deficit
• Microembolic events.

Quality of life

It is equally important to consider the physical and social impact of surgery—a patient may survive the procedure but never regain mobility or return to their previous independence and quality of life. Balancing this risk against current symptoms and quality of life is key to the decision making process and should involve both the patient and their relatives.

Perioperative care

The anaesthetist is responsible for the care of the patient from the time of induction of anaesthesia. Care during the first few postoperative days is often provided in conjunction with the surgical team.

Transoesophageal echocardiography is key in the perioperative period and may be performed by the anaesthetist, cardiologist, or a dedicated surgical echocardiography service.

Intra-operative transoesophageal echocardiography is strongly recommended during valve repair, surgery for IE and aortic valve surgery following dissection. It is also recommended during valve replacement although the evidence for improved outcomes in this setting is less robust. Potential application of transoesophageal echocardiography is broad but the following can be assessed:

• Baseline ventricular function
• Confirmation of pre-operative diagnosis
• Assessment of annular size
• Assessment of atheroma before cannulation of the aorta
• Position of atrial cannulae
• Air embolism—during de-airing
• Ventricular function following the procedure
• Results of valve intervention—residual regurgitation
• Exclusion of complications—e.g. systolic anterior motion of mitral valve.

Choice of surgery

The optimal surgical strategy is patient-specific and dictated by a large number of factors, including:

• Aetiology of valve lesion—primary or secondary valvular heart disease
• Underlying valve anatomy—bicuspid aortic valve?
• Dominant lesion—stenosis or regurgitation?
• Additional pathology—dilated aortic root?
• Need for concomitant bypass surgery
• Likelihood of durable repair
• Mechanical valve in another position?
• Risk of future IE or thromboembolic complications
• Contraindications to anticoagulation
• Biventricular function
• Comorbidities
• Possibility of future pregnancy
• Life expectancy.

This list is not exhaustive—many further issues will influence the planned procedure and choice of prosthetic valve if a repair cannot be achieved.

Types of prosthetic valve

Mechanical valves	
St Jude Medical	Bi-leaflet
CarboMedics®	Bi-leaflet carbon discs
Sorin Bicarbon™	Bi-leaflet carbon discs
Medtronic-Hall™	Single tilting disc
Bjork–Shiley	Single tilting disc
Starr–Edwards	Ball-in-cage
Mechanical composite	Mechanical valve with Dacron tube graft
Bioprosthetic valves	
Carpentier–Edwards®	Stented porcine valve
Medtronic (Hancock)	Stented modified porcine valve
Mosaic®	Stented porcine valve
Perimount	Stented bovine valve
Freestyle®	Stentless porcine aortic valve and root
Toronto SPV®	Stentless porcine valve with polyester coating
Homograft	
Prepared from homograft bank	Cryopreserved valve from disease-free cadaver
Autograft	
Ross procedure	Pulmonary valve transposed to aortic position and replaced with pulmonary homograft

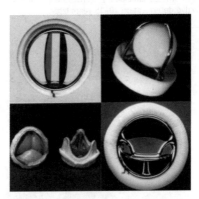

Fig.12.1 Variations in prosthetic valve design. Clockwise from top-left: St.Jude bi-leaflet, Starr–Edwards, Bjork–Shiley tilting disc, stented porcine bioprosthesis. Reproduced from Bloomfield P. (2002) Choice of heart valve prosthesis, *Heart*; 87:583–589 with permission from BMJ Publishing Group Ltd.

Mechanical vs. bioprosthetic valve (Fig. 12.1)

The choice of prosthesis is patient dependent and involves consideration of several factors which, including:

- Haemodynamic requirement—mechanical valves have better haemodynamic function than stented bioprostheses.
- Risk of anticoagulant related bleeding.
- Risk of valve deterioration.
- Life expectancy of the patient.

Factors favouring a mechanical prosthesis	Factors favouring a bioprosthesis
No contraindication to anticoagulation	Contraindication to anticoagulation
Increased risk of valve deterioration (young age, hyperparathyroidism, renal failure)	Poor compliance or lifestyle problems which may prevent safe anticoagulation (e.g. alcohol abuse)
Pre-existing requirement for anticoagulation	Patient preference (if appropriately informed) and low risk for future re-do surgery
Age <65 with no life limiting co-morbidities	Age >65–70 years or severe life-limiting comorbidity
High risk for re-do surgery (LV dysfunction, prior CABG, multivalve disease)	Prior mechanical valve thrombosis despite anticoagulation
Pre-existing mechanical prosthesis	Planned pregnancy

The emergence of transcatheter valve implantation may further alter current management strategies—for example, a patient aged 60 may choose a bioprosthesis, anticipating transcatheter valve replacement in the event of valve deterioration 10–15 years later.

Mechanical valve—advantages and disadvantages

The benefits of a mechanical valve include:
- Durable – lasts >30 years
- Haemodynamics—improved effective orifice area compared to some stented bioprostheses.

Principal drawbacks are:
- Need for life-long anticoagulation
- High trans-valvular gradients associated with small valves
- Loss of aortic annulus dynamics (fixed ring size and shape)
- Valve thrombosis even with adequate anticoagulation (0.2–5.7% per patient year)
- Higher risk of IE—3% at 1 year and 5.7% at 5 years
- Haemolysis—can lead to recurrent transfusion requirement
- Noise—may be intrusive or even intolerable
- Significant risks during pregnancy given need for anticoagulation (embryopathy, maternal and foetal bleeding).

Bioprosthetic valve—advantages and disadvantages

The main benefits of a bioprosthetic valve are:
- No need for life-long anticoagulation—thrombosis risk <1% per year
- Improved haemodynamics, especially with stentless bioprostheses.

Principal drawbacks include:
- Valve failure—>40% at 10 years
- Calcification—associated with progressive stenosis
- Implantation—technically more challenging, particularly using stentless valves
- IE—risk is higher than native valve but less than mechanical valve in the first 5 years after surgery.

Bioprosthetic mitral valves fail earlier than bioprosthetic aortic valves. Overall failure rate is around 60% at 15 years.

Aortic valve surgery

Techniques and routines vary considerably, but a typical aortic valve replacement procedure consists of the following steps:

- Midline sternotomy
- Standard cardiopulmonary bypass with 2-stage venous cannulae and heparin
- Antegrade cardioplegia—into aortic root (unless significant AR when direct cardioplegia into the coronary ostia or retrograde cardioplegia via the coronary sinus are used)
- Aortotomy
- Valve excision
- Decalcification of annulus
- Sizing of prosthesis
- Valve insertion—subcoronary or supra-annular
- Aortotomy closure
- De-airing—apical and aortic vents
- Weaning from bypass
- Protamine administration to reverse heparin
- Removal of venous and arterial cannulae
- Wire closure of sternotomy.

Additional options

- Sub-coronary stentless aortic valve implantation—a Medtronic Freestyle prosthesis or homograft can be tailored and sutured to the annulus. The porcine aorta sits inside the native aorta; sections of the prosthesis are removed to prevent obstruction of the native coronary ostia.
- Aortic root replacement— requiring isolation of the native coronary ostia as 'buttons' which are transferred to the prosthesis. The procedure is more demanding and time consuming.
- Cylinder technique—the prosthesis is prepared with coronary ostia created then implanted inside the native aorta.
- Ross procedure—a complex and challenging procedure to replace the aortic valve with the native pulmonary valve, which is in turn replaced with a pulmonary homograft.

Additional aortic root surgery

Depending on the anatomy and status of the aortic valve, a number of potential strategies are available:

- Aortic root and valve homograft
- Bentall procedure—a composite graft containing a mechanical aortic prosthesis in a Dacron tube—implantation requires mobilization of the native coronary ostia and re-implantation onto the graft
- Root enlargement—various techniques to avoid implantation of an excessively small prosthesis, usually involving division of the posterior aortic root and repair with a pericardial or Dacron patch
- Valve sparing root replacement—if AR is due to aortic disease, a variety of potential procedures can be performed to preserve the native aortic valve or re-suspend it within a graft.

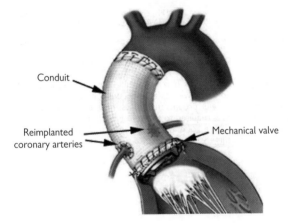

Conduit

Reimplanted coronary arteries

Mechanical valve

Fig. 12.2 Composite graft used in the Bentall procedure.

Classification of valve anatomy

A functional classification of aortic valve anatomy (similar to the Carpentier system for MR) has been devised to assist in the planning of surgery for AR.

Type	Pathology	Usual aetiology	Surgical option
Ia	Aneurysm of ascending aorta	Atherosclerotic degeneration	Remodel sinotubular junction
Ib	Aneurysm of aortic root	Marfan's syndrome	Remodelling or implantation technique
Ic	Isolated dilation of functional aortic annulus	Bicuspid valve disease	Partial subcommisural annuloplasty
Id	Perforation of leaflet	Infection or trauma	Pericardial patch
II	Leaflet prolapse	Hypertension or degeneration	Plication, resection or resuspension
III	Restrictive	Rheumatic disease	Not suitable for repair

Aortic valve repair

Selected patients with AR may be suitable for valve repair (Fig. 12.3), sparing the need for valve replacement with its attendant long-term complications. Careful preoperative assessment using transoesophageal echocardiography is required to assess lesion classification and suitability. Long term results are good, particularly in bicuspid aortic valve disease, with late re-do surgery required in <10% (Fig. 12.4).

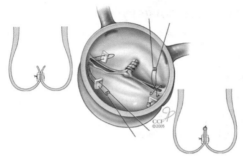

Fig. 12.3 Bicuspid aortic valve repair with Cabrol sutures, figure of 8 and leaflet placation. Reproduced with permission from Svensson L.G., Deglurkar I., and Ung J. (2007) Aortic Valve Repair and Root Preservation by Remodeling, Reimplantation, and Tailoring: Technical Aspects and Early Outcome *J Card Surg*. 22:473–479.

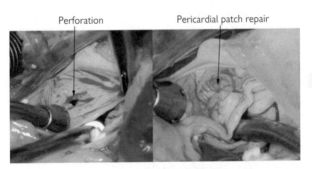

Perforation   Pericardial patch repair

Fig. 12.4 Pericardial patch repair for aortic valve perforation complicating IE. Reproduced with permission from ℘ http://www.ctsnet.org/sections/clinicalresources/adultcardiac/expert_tech-19.html. Copyright 2010 CTSNet, Inc. All rights reserved. Image is reproduced by permission of CTSNet, Inc.

Mitral valve surgery

Again, techniques are varied but a typical mitral valve repair will involve the following steps:
- Midline sternotomy
- Bi-caval cannulae
- Standard cardiopulmonary bypass with heparin
- Antegrade cardioplegia
- Horizontal left atriotomy—between superior pulmonary veins
- Valve inspection including annulus, chordae, leaflets and commissures
- Prolapse repair
- Chordal shortening, transfer or use of neo-chordae
- Annuloplasty ring (optional)
- Closure of atriotomy
- De-airing—through mitral valve
- Weaning from bypass
- Protamine administration to reverse heparin
- Removal of venous and arterial cannulae
- Wire closure of sternotomy.

In mitral valve replacement, the posterior leaflet and subvalvular apparatus are preserved to maintain normal LV wall stress and function.

Additional options

Valve replacement can also be performed in a number of alternative ways, although these are specialised and rarely used.
- Beating heart surgery—used to avoid damage to previous bypass grafts. The heart is left beating or fibrillating whilst on bypass
- Minimal access surgery—limited sternotomy incisions can be used for aortic valve surgery and thoracoscopic mitral valve repair and replacement has been performed.

Mitral valve repair

The optimal management of symptomatic severe MR is surgical valve repair, which carries a significantly lower morbidity and mortality than replacement surgery. Careful patient selection is crucial—only those in whom repair is not feasible should be referred for elective valve replacement.

Features favouring valve repair include:
• Limited segment of prolapse
• Minimal annular calcification
• Minimal leaflet calcification
• Absence of rheumatic disease or leaflet thickening
• Normal annular size.

Appropriate imaging to demonstrate the mechanism of MR is vital to identify suitability for repair. While repair of isolated posterior segment prolapse is relatively straightforward, anterior leaflet prolapse with associated chordal disease is much more challenging and requires considerable surgical expertise. In Europe, valve repair is undertaken in approximately 50% of patients requiring mitral valve surgery. One third of the patients who receive a mechanical valve do so due to a lack of local expertise in valve repair.

Published recommendations for establishing a dedicated mitral valve repair service include:
• At least 50 repair procedures/year, each individual surgeon performing >25/year after specific training
• Dedicated cardiologist with subspecialist interest in valvular heart disease
• High quality intra-operative transoesophageal echocardiography by accredited cardiologists or anaesthetists
• Additional expertise in surgical ablation of atrial fibrillation
• Multidisciplinary mitral valve team to allow appropriate case selection
• Audit of activity and outcomes
• Mortality for isolated repair <1% and 5 year re-operation rate <5%.

(Bridgewater B., Hooper T., Munsch C. et al. (2006) Heart 92:939–944).

Methods of repair

Various techniques have been described. Surgical repair requires a comprehensive approach to all aspects of the mitral valve complex to achieve valve competence with a large coaptation area but no prolapse.

The goals of mitral valve repair are:
• Restoration of the proper line of coaptation of both leaflets
• Preservation or restoration of full leaflet motion
• Correction of annular dilation
• Preservation of subvalvar apparatus
• Minimal or no residual MR.

Pathology	Main technique	Additional options
Posterior prolapse	Quadrangular excision and annuloplasty ring	Chordal shortening or resection Sliding leaflet plasty
Anterior prolapse	Triangular resection and annuloplasty ring	Chordal transfer Artificial chordae
Bileaflet prolapse	Posterior leaflet resection and annuloplasty ring	Alfieri stitch Sliding leaflet plasty
Annular dilation	Annuloplasty ring	
Papillary rupture	Papillary reimplantation	

Leaflet resection

Excessive leaflet tissue is resected and the cut edges sutured to reduce their width and height. Quadrangular resection is performed in the most common scenario of P2 segment prolapse. Sliding plasty refers to more extensive resection of excess tissue and re-approximation of the free edges (Fig. 12.5).

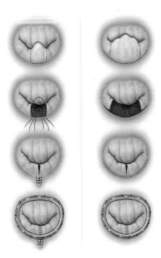

Fig. 12.5 The left hand panel shows repair of isolated P2 prolapse by quadrangular resection followed by annuloplasty. The right hand panel shows repair of excessive posterior leaflet tissue by resection and sliding plasty followed by annuloplasty. Reproduced with permission from Verma S., Mesana T.G. (2009) Mitral-Valve Repair for Mitral-Valve Prolapse *NEJM* 361:2261–2269. Copyright 2009 Massachusetts Medical Society. All rights reserved.

Annuloplasty ring

The function of the ring is to reduce annular diameter and suture tension while maintaining flexibility and normal motion throughout the cardiac cycle. Early rigid annuloplasty rings have now been replaced by flexible devices which mimic normal annular geometry (Fig. 12.6).

Anticoagulation is usually required for three months following surgery (or longer if other indications exist e.g. atrial fibrillation).

Chordal transfer and use of neo-chordae

An intact chord inserting into a normal segment of the mitral valve can be detached and reimplanted onto a prolapsed segment. Alternatively, artificial chords, usually made of polytetrafluoroethylene, can be used to join the prolapsing edge and relevant papillary muscle (Fig. 12.7).

The older technique of chordal shortening (splitting the papillary muscle and re-embedding the chordae) is now less frequently used due to concerns for papillary muscle blood supply.

Alfieri stitch

A suture joining the free leaflet edges creates a double orifice mitral valve and relative MS, but is effective at reducing MR. The procedure is no longer commonly used but has spawned a percutaneous technique using a similar principle (Fig. 12.8).

Papillary reimplantation

In patients with ischaemic papillary muscle rupture it may be possible to re-attach the fibrous tip of the muscle to an adjacent viable segment.

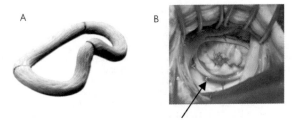

Fig. 12.6 (A) Edwards Geoform ring (B) implanted annuloplasty ring.
Fig. 12.6 (A) Reproduced with permission from Edwards Lifesciences, Irvine
California. Fig. 12.6 (B) Reproduced with permission from Al-Attar N. (2008)
Infective Endocarditis E-Journal of the ESC Council for Cardiology Practice 7; 5
(31st Dec 2008)
🖰 http://www.edwards.com/products/rings/geoform.htm and ESC website
🖰 http://www.escardio.org/communities/councils/ccp/e-journal/volume7/pages/
infective-endocarditis.aspx respectively. See also **Plate 19**.

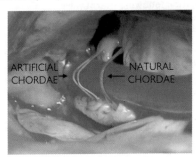

Fig. 12.7 Surgically implanted artificial chordae with natural chordae alongside
for comparison. Reproduced from Salvador, L *et al* (2008). A 20-year experience with
mitral valve repair with artificial chordae in 608 patients J Thorac Cardiovasc Surg
2008; 135: 1280–1287, with permission from Elsevier. From website 🖰 http://www.
westernthoracic.org/Abstracts/2007/9.html. See also **Plate 20**.

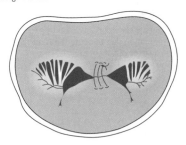

Fig. 12.8 The Alfieri stitch which opposes the anterior and posterior leaflets to
create a double orifice mitral valve.

Management following mitral valve repair

The competence of the repair is confirmed visually and challenged by distending the LV with saline injected through the mitral valve. Once the patient has been weaned from cardiopulmonary bypass, the degree of any MR should be assessed using transoesophageal echocardiography. It is imperative this assessment is performed under 'normal' haemodynamic conditions—inotropes and vasopressors should be used to simulate expected postoperative blood pressure and filling conditions.

The restoration of mitral valve competence leads to an abrupt increase in LV afterload. Patients, particularly those with pre-existing LV dysfunction, may require intensive support with inotropes, intra-aortic balloon pump, pacing therapy and vasodilators. In extreme cases LV assist devices may be used to bridge the patient to recovery.

Patients should undergo transthoracic echocardiography before discharge to document mitral valve, LV and RV function with re-assessment at eight weeks. Annual surveillance with clinical review and echocardiography is recommended thereafter.

Anticoagulation following mitral valve repair

If a patient has undergone a standard mitral valve repair (including annuloplasty) and is in sinus rhythm then aspirin alone is sufficient thromboprophylaxis. If the patient has experienced post operative atrial fibrillation or has a high thromboembolic risk then anticoagulation (INR 2.0–2.5) is recommended for at least three months.

Complications of mitral valve repair

The reported mortality following mitral valve repair is 1–2% when performed in high-volume centres.

Adverse events during the postoperative period can include:
- Heart failure—the most common cause of mortality
- Renal failure—2–3%
- Stroke—1%
- Repeat operation—6%
- MS—rare but can occur if annuloplasty is undersized
- Damage to circumflex coronary artery
- Damage to conduction system
- Haemolysis, often related to high velocity jet of residual MR through small remaining orifice.

Around 5–10% of patients require conversion to mitral valve replacement at the time of first operation due to acute failure of their repair. Late MR occurs in up to one quarter of patients.

Systolic anterior motion

Postoperative systolic anterior motion of the mitral valve (SAM) is reported in ~5% of repair procedures and can lead to outflow tract obstruction and haemodynamic compromise, particularly if perioperative inotropes are used (Fig. 12.9).

The risk of postoperative SAM is increased by several anatomical factors:
• Elongated anterior leaflet
• Anterior papillary muscles
• Non-dilated LV
• Narrow angle between aortic and mitral valves
• Anterior-posterior leaflet ratio <1
• Anterior coaptation point
• Distance between coaptation point and septum <2.5cm.

If highlighted before surgery, the operative strategy can be modified. Annuloplasty may increase the antero-posterior diameter and sliding plasty of the posterior leaflet will increase the distance between the coaptation point and the septum.

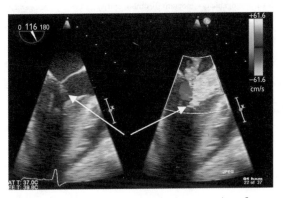

Fig. 12.9 Postoperative SAM—the anterior leaflet deviates into the outflow tract during systole with resultant flow obstruction (highlighted with colour Doppler—arrowed). These changes resolved with increased filling pressures and reduced inotropic support. See also **Plate 21**.

Anticoagulation

Oral anticoagulation is commenced in the early postoperative period if haemostasis is secure and all drains have been removed.

Oral anticoagulation is recommended in:
• All mechanical prostheses—lifelong therapy with warfarin (or alternative vitamin K antagonist)
• Bioprosthesis with increased embolic risk—atrial fibrillation, heart failure
• Bioprosthesis for 3 months—many use aspirin instead of warfarin.

The risk of thromboembolism is highest in the early postoperative period, so appropriate arrangements for close monitoring of the INR are required.

The risk of thromboembolism is dependent on the combination of valve type, prosthesis position, and patient related factors. The inherent degree of thrombogenicity varies with valve type:

Low thrombogenicity	Medium thrombogenicity	High thrombogenicity
CarboMedics valve	Bjork–Shiley valve	Omniscience
Medtronic Hall	Other bi-leaflet valves	Starr–Edwards
St. Jude Medical		

Additional risk factors when judging appropriate anticoagulation include:

Prosthesis factors	Patient factors
Mitral > aortic (lower flow velocity)	Previous thromboembolism, thrombophilia
Smaller diameter valve	Atrial fibrillation
Right sided mechanical prostheses > left sided	Large left atrium, dense spontaneous echo contrast
Multiple prostheses	Ejection fraction <35%

Recommended level of anticoagulation

A patient-specific judgement based on the above factors is required to guide appropriate anticoagulation. As an approximate guide, the following mean INR should be recommended:

	Associated risk factors	
Prosthesis thrombogenicity	Absent	Present
Low	INR 2.5	INR 3.0
Medium	INR 3.0	INR 3.5
High	INR 3.5	INR 4.0

Valve thrombosis

Prosthetic valve thrombosis is a feared complication which is fortunately rare. Bioprosthetic valves and homografts may be affected but in 95% a mechanical prosthesis is involved. The overall rate of thrombosis of mechanical prostheses is between 0.3–1.3% per patient year.

The main cause of valve thrombosis is failure of anticoagulation which may be caused by:
- Cessation of treatment
- Poor compliance
- Interaction with new medication—e.g. antibiotic therapy
- Intercurrent illness—dehydration, infection
- Hypercoagulable state—malignancy, surgery.

The possibility of valve thrombosis should be considered in any patient with a prosthetic valve who develops:
- Shortness of breath
- Fatigue
- Cardiac failure
- Systemic embolism.

These symptoms may develop acutely or gradually over days to weeks. Evidence of a period of sub-optimal anticoagulation greatly increases the likelihood of thrombosis.

Thrombosis often develops on pre-existent fibrous pannus—such fibrous in-growth over the valve is found in up to three quarters of patients presenting with valve thrombosis.

Investigation of suspected valve thrombosis

Clinical assessment including a history and physical examination should pay particular attention to a detailed drug history, recent INR readings and doses and the introduction of any new medication. The patient should be challenged on compliance and the dose regime verified.

Physical signs relate to the prosthesis position—left sided valve thrombosis (the most common scenario) usually causes pulmonary oedema and poor systemic perfusion. Indistinct prosthetic heart sounds may be a subtle sign of prosthetic valve failure, and a new obstructive or regurgitant murmur may also be heard.

Definitive diagnosis requires imaging. Fluoroscopy is a rapid method to assess mechanical valve function which may easily identify a fixed leaflet or asymmetrical leaflet motion (Fig. 12.10).

Echocardiography may also assess valve appearance, leaflet motion and trans-valvular gradient. Often a combination of transthoracic and transoesophageal imaging is required. Prosthetic mitral valves are easier to image than aortic prostheses, since a large left atrium facilitates views of the mitral valve.

In borderline cases, comparison with baseline or recent echocardiographic studies can be help to document clear changes in prosthetic function and support the diagnosis of valve thrombosis.

Suspicious prosthetic valve Doppler data

The gradient through the prosthesis depends on its size and type. As an approximate guide, prosthetic obstruction should be suspected if the following are detected:

- Mitral prosthesis with mean gradient >8mmHg and effective orifice area <1.3cm^2
- Aortic prosthesis with mean gradient >45mmHg.

Management of prosthetic valve thrombosis

The only therapeutic options for prosthetic valve thrombosis are valve replacement or thrombolysis. A patient with suspected or proven valve thrombosis should receive immediate anticoagulation with intravenous heparin and be transferred to a cardiothoracic surgical centre.

The default treatment in patients with severe symptoms and thrombosis of a mitral or aortic prosthesis should be re-do valve replacement surgery. Rescue thrombolysis may be considered in:

• Critical haemodynamic state but excessive risk for re-do valve replacement surgery
• High likelihood of death before surgery is available.

Thrombolysis is not without risk—20% of patients will develop a systemic embolism and 20% will re-thrombose the valve. Furthermore, major bleeding occurs in around 5%.

Thrombolysis is a more successful treatment option in patients with thrombosis of a tricuspid or pulmonary prosthesis.

If a patient is haemodynamically stable then intensified anticoagulation (initially with intravenous heparin then higher dose warfarin) may be sufficient for thrombus regression—close monitoring and serial imaging are required.

If prosthetic valve thrombosis develops despite apparently adequate anticoagulation then screening for thrombophilia is appropriate. Adjustment of the target INR or additional anti-platelet therapy (e.g. aspirin) are potential treatment strategies.

Thrombolysis protocols

There is no evidence base to guide thrombolysis regimes and various protocols have been suggested.

Rescue thrombolysis for critically ill patients unsuitable for surgery or unlikely to survive transfer should comprise:
- Tissue plasminogen activator (tPA)—10mg bolus then 90mg over 90 minutes

or
- 1.5 million units Streptokinase over 60 minutes.

In a haemodynamically stable patient, thrombolysis may be delivered over a longer period, for example:
- Tissue plasminogen activator (tPA)—10mg bolus then 50mg in first hour and 20mg per hour for two hours.

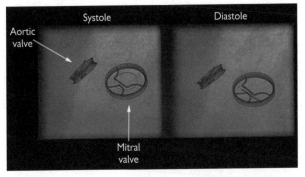

Fig. 12.10 Systolic and diastolic frames in a patient with mechanical aortic and mitral valves. Note how the occluder of the aortic valve does not move (arrowed) strongly suggesting valve thrombosis.

Thromboembolism

A thromboembolic event in a patient with a prosthetic valve does not directly implicate the valve—many patients have additional risk factors (such as atrial fibrillation).

While it is tempting to assume inadequate anticoagulation and recommend a higher mean INR, any patient with a prosthetic valve who sustains a thromboembolic event should undergo through assessment to identify or exclude alternative causes:

- Assessment of recent anticoagulation and compliance
- Examination—new murmur or muffled valve sounds?
- IE screen—blood cultures, temperature and inflammatory markers
- ECG—new atrial fibrillation?
- Blood glucose—new diabetes mellitus?
- Carotid Doppler—carotid atheroma?
- Transthoracic and transoesophageal echocardiography (Fig. 12.11)
- Fluoroscopy of valve leaflets.

A cerebrovascular thromboembolic event must be evaluated with imaging to exclude intra-cranial haemorrhage. Magnetic resonance imaging is safe in patients with mechanical prostheses.

Management of thromboembolism

Treatment is directed at the cause—e.g. treatment of hypertension and diabetes.

If thromboembolism related to a prosthetic valve is suspected and no other cause identified then the options include:

- Intensified anticoagulant therapy—increase target mean INR by 0.5
- Add aspirin 75mg to warfarin.

Balancing these options against the increased risk of bleeding can be challenging, particularly if there has been a recent cerebrovascular event.

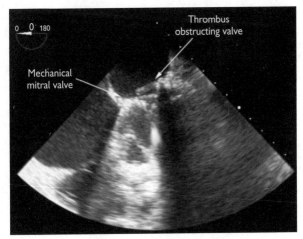

Fig. 12.11 Thrombus in the left atrium demonstrated on transthoracic echocardiography in a patient with a mechanical mitral valve prosthesis.

Bleeding or INR elevation

The risk of bleeding on warfarin is related to the level of INR. Major bleeding risk increases when the INR is >4.5, with a more rapid increase in risk when >6.0.

If a patient's INR is greater than 6.0, management is guided by the presence or absence of bleeding.

Management of INR elevation without bleeding

If the INR is >6.0 and the patient is not actively bleeding management should consist of:

• Admission to hospital
• Discontinuation of warfarin
• Close monitoring of INR
• Re-introduction of warfarin when INR is <5.0
• Careful monitoring to ensure INR does not undershoot target
• Heparin cover if INR falls below target.

If the INR is >10.0, fresh frozen plasma (FFP) can be infused to reduce the INR. However, FFP does not contain sufficient concentration of Vitamin K dependent clotting factors (notably Factor IX) to fully reverse the bleeding tendency. A dose of 15ml/Kg is usually recommended.

Vitamin K administration in high doses leads to rapid and prolonged reversal of warfarin and may cause valve thrombosis or micro-embolism. Therefore, small doses (0.5–1.0mg preferably IV) are recommended for the reversal of an elevated INR.

Management of INR elevation with bleeding

The appropriate management of a patient with a prosthetic valve and a major bleed associated with an elevated INR depends on the balance of risks. Intracranial and major gastro-intestinal bleeding requires rapid and complete reversal of anticoagulation.

This is best achieved with:
- Intravenous prothrombin complex concentrate (PCC)—30units/kg
- Intravenous fresh frozen plasma if PCC not available—15ml/kg
- Intravenous vitamin K 5mg if bleeding continues

Similarly decision-making on the reintroduction of anticoagulation— usually beginning with intravenous heparin depends on the cause of the bleed and whether a preventative intervention has been performed.

Intracerebral haemorrhage is a particularly difficult complication to manage—limited guidance exists but consideration of re-anticoagulation at one week is reasonable, depending on the thrombogenicity of the valve and previous thromboembolic events.

Haemolysis

Haemolytic anaemia may occur with mechanical and bioprotheses, and even after mitral valve repair. It is a rare finding and should prompt screening for mechanical valve dysfunction or a paravalvular leak.

Chronic mild haemolysis without clinical sequelae is comparatively common. However, anaemia requiring recurrent transfusion is rare and more likely to occur in patients with older or multiple mechanical valves.

Evidence for anaemia due to haemolysis includes:
• Persistent anaemia (Hb<10g/dl)
• Elevated lactate dehydrogenase >440U/L
• Reduced serum haptoglobin
• Schistocytes and fragmented cells on blood film
• Increased reticulocyte count
• Increased urinary urobilinogen.

If haemolysis is identified and no alternative cause found then valve assessment using echocardiography (+/– fluoroscopy) is required (Fig. 12.12).

Management of haemolysis

Haemolytic anaemia leads to increased cardiac output and reduced blood viscosity which may further increase haemolysis. Supplemental iron and folate are required along with transfusion to maintain the haemoglobin above the level at which symptoms develop.

Re-do surgery may be required for severe intractable haemolysis. If paravalvular leak is the underlying cause then percutaneous treatment may be feasible (See 📖 p.295).

Medical management is limited—β-blockers reduce the frequency of red cell trauma in some patients and erythropoietin can be useful to maintain adequate haemoglobin levels.

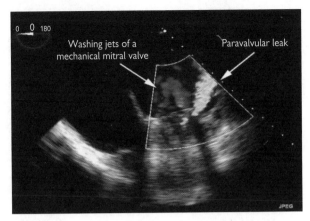

Fig. 12.12 Transoesophageal echocardiogram of a paraprosthetic leak—this narrow high velocity jet was causing persistent haemolysis. See also **Plate 22**.

Paravalvular leak

Significant paravalvular leak is an uncommon complication of valve replacement and should always prompt a thorough search for IE. Small incidental leaks are seen in 5% of aortic valve replacements and 10% of mitral valve replacements.

A heavily-calcified annulus at the time of surgery may prevent circumferential seating of the prosthesis and cause a chronic paravalvular leak. Haemolysis, heart failure, and progressive LV dysfunction may result.

Re-do surgery is required in selected patients, although many paravalvular leaks may be amenable to percutaneous closure (if IE has been excluded). A specific size and shaped device is delivered across the leak using a retrograde or antegrade approach (Fig. 12.13 & Fig. 12.14). The presence of the device itself reduces the leak significantly, although subsequent endothelial formation and fibrosis further abolish flow.

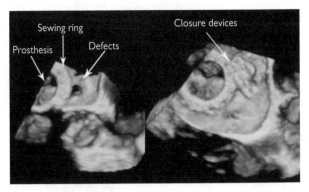

Fig. 12.13 3D transoesophageal imaging. The left hand panel shows a mitral bioprosthesis with two defects around the sewing ring. The right hand panel demonstrates the final appearance of two occluder devices deployed across the defect to abolish the MR. See also **Plate 23**.

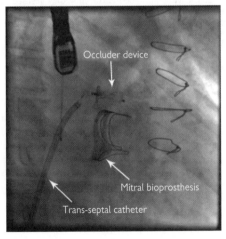

Fig. 12.14 Fluoroscopic image of first occluder delivered via a trans-septal approach.

Bioprosthetic failure

Modern bioprosthetic valves are durable, with 70% of aortic bioprotheses free of any evidence of structural deterioration at 5 years. Mitral bioprosthesis have less durability and only 40% have no structural decline at 5 years.

Ultimately around 30% of bioprosthetic valves require re-intervention 10–15 years after implantation because of structural failure, usually due to rupture of a diseased calcified cusp with severe regurgitation (Fig. 12.15). Rarely, calcific stenosis develops.

The patient usually reports gradual development of the symptoms of heart failure. Symptoms may be initially controlled with medical therapy allowing intervention to be delayed or deferred.

The rate of structural failure is inversely related to the age of the patient at the time of implantation—40% of prostheses implanted into patients <40 years of age fail within 10 years, compared to only 10% of those implanted in patients >70 years of age.

Many patients are unsuitable for re-do valve surgery due to advanced age and comorbidities. In younger patients, re-do surgery is appropriate following careful discussion concerning the choice of prosthesis.

Transcatheter valve implantation is currently only licensed for native AS but limited reports of its use for the treatment of failing aortic bioprostheses in elderly patients have emerged—the so called 'valve-in-valve' technique.

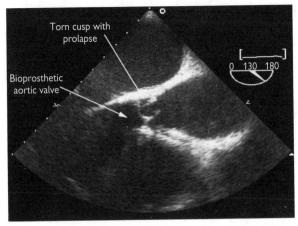

Fig. 12.15 Severe aortic regurgitation due to failure of a bioprosthetic aortic valve and cusp prolapse.

Patient–prosthesis mismatch

The term patient–prosthesis mismatch is used to describe the effect of implantation of a prosthesis with an effective orifice area which is too small in relation to the patient's body size.

The net effect is a higher than expected gradient across a normally functioning prosthesis.

Mismatch is defined by indexing the effective orifice area of the prosthesis to the patient's body surface area, with a recommended cut-off of <0.85cm^2/m^2. An indexed orifice area <0.65cm^2/m^2 suggests severe patient-prosthesis mismatch.

Rates of moderate mismatch are 20–70% but severe mismatch is seen in only 2–11% of patients, most frequently in those with an aortic prosthesis.

Diagnosis

The effective orifice area of the prosthesis cannot be derived from knowledge of the valve size and type. Manufacturers do provide the internal geometric area of all prosthetic valves, but this figure bears no relation to postoperative haemodynamic function.

The effective orifice area is therefore derived using echocardiography and the continuity equation (See 📖 p.62) The patient's height and weight are used to calculate body surface area (BSA):

$$BSA = \sqrt{\frac{height(cm) \times weight(kg)}{3600}}$$

The effective orifice area is divided by the body surface are to provide an indexed value.

Exercise echocardiography

If there is discordance between a patient's symptoms and the resting echocardiographic assessment, monitoring the transvalvular gradient during exercise may unmask significant patient–prosthesis mismatch. If the transvalvular gradient increases by >20mmHg for aortic prostheses or >12mmHg for mitral prostheses then mismatch should be suspected.

Implications

Patient–prosthesis mismatch leads to reduced regression of LV mass and remodelling following surgery, and significant reduction in cardiac index during the early postoperative phase. Early mortality is higher in patients with severe mismatch, with additional evidence of increased late morality—perhaps due to less effective orifice area 'reserve'.

Prevention

The minimum effective orifice area to prevent mismatch can be derived by calculating the patient's body surface area and multiplying by $0.85 \text{cm}^2/\text{m}^2$. The appropriate prosthesis size can then be chosen based on the reference values for effective orifice area.

Valve type	19mm	21mm	23mm	25mm	27mm	29mm
Stented bioprosthesis						
Medtronic Mosaic®	1.20	1.22	1.38	1.65	1.80	2.00
Hancock II	NA	1.18	1.33	1.46	1.55	1.60
Perimount	1.10	1.30	1.50	1.80	1.80	NA
Stentless bioprosthesis						
Medtronic Freestyle®	1.15	1.35	1.48	2.00	2.32	NA
St Jude Toronto	–	1.30	1.50	1.70	2.00	2.50
Edwards Prima	0.80	1.10	1.50	1.80	2.30	2.80
Mechanical valves						
Medtronic Hall	1.19	1.34	NA	NA	NA	NA
St Jude Standard	1.04	1.38	1.52	2.08	2.65	3.23
St Jude Regent	1.60	2.00	2.20	2.50	3.60	4.40
CarboMedics®	1.00	1.54	1.63	1.98	2.41	2.63
Sorin Bicarbon™	NA	1.66	1.96	NA	NA	NA

Mean effective orifice area for commonly available prosthetic valves—modified from Pibarot and Dumesnil.

If mismatch is anticipated—e.g. if a small annulus prevents implantation of a larger valve, then options include:
• Use of a different prosthesis with a larger orifice area at that size
• Use of a homograft
• Enlargement of the aortic root during implantation.

Surveillance

Patients should be followed up early after prosthetic valve implantation to allow baseline assessment against which future assessments can be compared.

This visit should include
- Assessment of symptomatic status
- Documentation of physical signs and auscultation findings
- ECG
- Chest X-ray
- Transthoracic echocardiogram—gradients and effective orifice area
- Haematology to exclude anaemia.

Subsequent follow up will depend on the status of the patient and their prosthesis. Many centres advocate annual assessment of patients following valve surgery, with echocardiographic assessment in the event of changing symptoms or physical signs.

Routine annual echocardiography is not recommended unless:
- Known paravalvular leak
- Previous IE
- Previous valve thrombosis
- Bioprosthetic valve reaching end of expected durability
- Marfan's patient—to assess aortic root and mitral valve
- Coexistent native valve disease which may require further treatment.

Prosthetic valves in pregnancy

The key impact of a prosthetic valve during pregnancy is the need for continuous anticoagulation and increased risk of thrombosis. Co-ordinated collaboration between the cardiologist, obstetrician, haematologist, and patient is required. Maternal mortality during pregnancy with a prosthetic valve is 1–4% with most deaths occurring due to thromboembolic complications.

Warfarin risks teratogenicity (1st trimester), foetal haemorrhage (especially in 3rd trimester), and foetal loss throughout pregnancy. Heparin has been implicated in prosthetic valve thrombosis and may cause osteoporosis and thrombocytopenia if use is prolonged. Twice daily administration of low molecular weight heparin is preferred to unfractionated heparin—anti-Xa levels can be monitored and the longer half life results in more stable therapeutic levels.

General advice

The interests of the mother and foetus are in conflict and there is no perfect regime—the choice remains the subject of controversy in the specialist literature.

The three main options are:
• Low molecular weight heparin plus aspirin throughout pregnancy
• Warfarin throughout pregnancy, changing to unfractionated heparin at 36 weeks
• Low molecular weight heparin plus aspirin in 1st trimester, changing to warfarin until 36 weeks when unfractionated heparin is recommended.

Baseline examination (including echocardiography) should be performed as soon as pregnancy is apparent to document valve function and cardiac status, and exclude valve related complications.

Anticoagulation regimes and complication rates

Low molecular weight heparin is unlicensed for use in pregnant women with prosthetic valves and may carry a higher risk of valve thrombosis; it should be used with caution and frequent monitoring of anti-Xa activity. Warfarin is potentially teratogenic although the risk is extremely small if the daily dose is <5mg.

Possible combinations include:

Strategy	Foetal complications	Maternal complications
Low molecular weight heparin throughout	24% spontaneous abortion 0% embryopathy	33% thromboembolism 15% mortality
Low molecular weight heparin for first trimester and from week 36 with Warfarin in-between	24% spontaneous abortion 3% embryopathy	9% thromboembolism 4% mortality
Warfarin until week 36 then heparin	24% spontaneous abortion 6% embryopathy	4% thromboembolism 2% mortality

Given the high complication rates many experts advise use of warfarin at the lowest possible dose throughout pregnancy until week 36, followed by subcutaneous unfractionated heparin until delivery. Twice daily low molecular weight heparin maintaining a 4 hour post dose anti-Xa level of 0.7–1.2 U/ml is an alternative.

Management during delivery

Pregnancy confers relative heparin resistance, and careful monitoring of anticoagulant level is required.

Heparin is stopped when labour begins and restarted 4–6 hours after delivery. Warfarin is re-commenced after 24 hours.

If unexpected labour occurs while the patient is still taking Warfarin, the safest option is caesarean section with an INR of 2.0 to reduce the risk of foetal intra-cranial haemorrhage during vaginal delivery.

Magnetic resonance imaging and prosthetic valves

Almost all prosthetic heart valves are safe in a magnetic resonance imaging (MRI) scanner with a field strength of 1.5 Tesla. Most are also safe at 3 Tesla although formal test data are limited.

Many prostheses contain no ferro-magnetic components, but even in those that do the forces exerted on the valve during an MRI scan are negligible compared to the intrinsic forces during each cardiac cycle. A metallic prosthesis does produce artefact, but this is generally limited and rarely impacts on scanning (Fig. 12.16).

MRI scans can be useful in patients with prosthetic valves to assess:
- Regurgitant flow—valvular or paravalvular
- Flow pattern and velocity through the valve
- Leaflet motion
- LV and RV function.

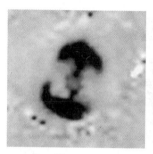 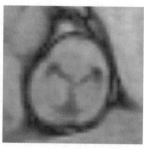

Fig. 12.16 Left hand panel shows a bileaflet tilting disc prosthesis with characteristic flow pattern through its orifices. Right hand panel shows an aortic bioprosthesis in diastole.

Percutaneous valve therapy

Introduction

Percutaneous treatment of MS has been available for over two decades and has now been followed by the introduction of percutaneous aortic and pulmonary valve implantation. Emerging technologies have allowed the recent development of a variety of percutaneous techniques to treat MR.

Percutaneous treatment of valvular heart disease has the potential to relieve symptoms in patients for whom conventional surgery presents excessive risk. It may also avoid surgical treatment altogether if ventricular dysfunction or other complications can be prevented.

Balloon mitral valvuloplasty

The use of a specialized balloon, delivered across the mitral valve via the atrial septum, and inflated to split the fused commissures in MS was first described in 1984. Short and medium term outcomes of the procedure are similar to those of surgical commissurotomy; despite obvious advantages for the patient, it is a complex and difficult procedure with a steep learning curve, and should only be performed in specialist centres by experienced operators.

Most patients achieve a doubling in mitral valve area and a 50–60% reduction in valve gradient. Complications include:
- Severe MR (2–10%)
- Residual atrial septal defect
- LV perforation
- Systemic embolism
- Death (< 1% in high volume centres).

Long term outcomes are favourable with 65% survival over 3–7 years, the vast majority (90%) of patients remaining in NYHA class I/II.

Patient selection
Indications and contraindications for balloon mitral valvuloplasty:

* (See 📖 p.168).

Indications	Contraindications
Symptomatic patient	Asymptomatic unless high risk clinical features
Mitral valve area <1.5cm^2	Left atrial thrombus
Wilkins score <8	Moderate MR
Favourable valve anatomy	Wilkins score >8
High risk of decompensation	Prior valvuloplasty (relative)
Desire for pregnancy	Alternative indication for cardiac surgery

Technique

The procedure is carried out using fluoroscopy and echocardiographic guidance. General anaesthesia and continuous transoesophageal monitoring or light sedation with transthoracic echocardiography are equally feasible according to operator preference and expertise. The use of intracardiac echocardiography has also been described recently.

The atrial septum is crossed following access from the femoral vein (Fig. 13.1) and a specialized (Inoue) balloon passed through the stenosed mitral valve. The balloon inflates sequentially: the distal then proximal portions initially expand to secure the balloon's position across the valve before final expansion of the central section applies force to the leaflet tips and splits the commissures (Fig. 13.2).

Stepwise inflations with steadily increasing balloon diameters are undertaken and results assessed at each stage using echocardiography. Valve area is assessed by planimetry with careful monitoring for the development of MR (Fig.13.3).

Following the procedure, patients require early re-assessment to ensure symptomatic improvement and echocardiographic integrity of the result. Re-stenosis occurs rarely and annual long-term follow-up is recommended.

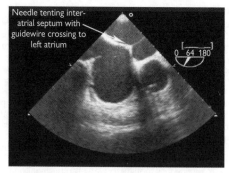

Fig. 13.1 Transoesophageal echocardiogram during trans-septal puncture.

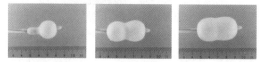

Fig. 13.2 The steps of balloon inflation. From Toray USA website ℘ www.ptmv. org/instrballoon.htm.

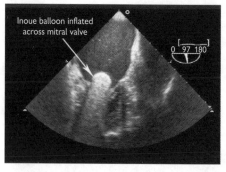

Fig.13.3 Transoesophageal echocardiogram demonstrating Inoue balloon inflation across the mitral valve.

Percutaneous treatment of mitral regurgitation

Historically, MR could only be relieved by surgical repair (or replacement if not feasible) but a number of percutaneous approaches have been recently developed and are now entering clinical practice.

Edge-to-edge repair

Designed to mimic the Alfieri stitch repair, available technologies include a deployable clip (Fig. 13.4) which grasps the leaflets, and a suction suture device, both delivered via trans-septal puncture. The procedure is performed under general anaesthesia and transoesophageal echocardiographic guidance. Preliminary clinical experience suggests the procedure is safe and feasible with reduction in the degree of MR and good clinical outcomes. Controlled trials are ongoing.

Coronary sinus annuloplasty

The coronary sinus runs adjacent to the posterior mitral annulus and a variety of devices have been designed for deployment within it to induce changes in annular size and shape with consequent reduction in MR (Fig. 13.5). Favourable initial results await further assessment in ongoing clinical trials. Variation in the anatomy of the coronary sinus and its relation to the mitral annulus and concern over compression of the adjacent circumflex coronary artery may limit this approach.

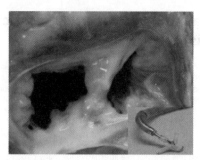

Fig. 13.4 Results 6 months after deployment of an Evalve clip in a porcine model. Reproduced from Coats, Bonhoeffer (2007) New percutaneous treatments for heart disease, *Heart*; 93:639–644) with permission of BMJ Publishing Group Ltd. See also **Plate 24**.

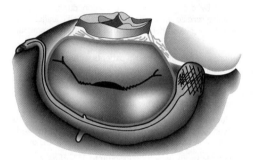

Fig. 13.5 The Edwards Monarch system—a shaped constraining device deployed in the coronary sinus. See also **Plate 25**.

Percutaneous treatment of aortic stenosis

Introduction

Percutaneous treatment of AS is not a new concept. Balloon aortic valvuloplasty was developed over 20 years ago as an option for patients unsuitable for conventional aortic valve surgery, but fell into disrepute as a result of high complication rates and poor long term outcomes. The emergence of transcatheter aortic valve implantation (TAVI) in the past five years has brought about a resurgence of interest in this area—both balloon valvuloplasty and TAVI relieve symptoms of AS and rapidly evolving technical advances make this an attractive alternative for many patients.

Balloon aortic valvuloplasty

The procedure involves passage of a guidewire across the stenosed aortic valve followed by progressive balloon dilation during rapid ventricular pacing (achieving cardiac standstill) to fracture calcific leaflet deposits and expand the valve annulus: there is minimal impact on commissural fusion (Fig. 13.6).

The procedure may be considered in patients with:
- Critically unstable symptoms (often as a bridge to surgery)
- Symptomatic severe AS and need for urgent non-cardiac surgery
- Contraindications to surgical valve replacement
- Severe symptomatic AS in pregnancy.

Modest reductions in peak and mean gradients are usually obtained. However, even a small increase in valve area can lead to marked symptomatic improvement, which may be sustained for 12 months or more.

Significant complications (which occur in up to 25% of patients) include:
- Cardiac tamponade
- Acute AR
- Arrhythmia
- Myocardial infarction
- Systemic embolism (including stroke)
- Access site complications.

The procedure does not alter the natural history of severe AS. Although rapid re-stenosis is uncommon, 20% of elderly patients have significant re-stenosis at 12 months. Repeated procedures are feasible but seldom appropriate. The combination of aortic valvuloplasty and percutaneous coronary intervention for symptom relief in patients with severe AS and coronary artery disease has been reported with encouraging results.

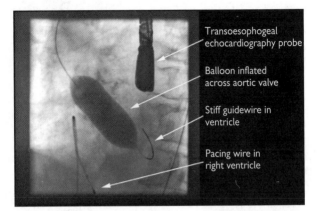

Transoesophogeal echocardiography probe

Balloon inflated across aortic valve

Stiff guidewire in ventricle

Pacing wire in right ventricle

Fig. 13.6 Balloon aortic valvuloplasty under transoesophageal echocardiographic guidance—the inflation is performed during rapid ventricular pacing to reduce cardiac output and ensure a stable balloon position.

Transcatheter aortic valve implantation

The first percutaneous implantation of a balloon-expanded aortic valve prosthesis was performed in 2002. Technically the native valve is not replaced but excluded by the prosthesis (Fig. 13.7). Furthermore, not all approaches are truly percutaneous, hence the preferred term of TAVI. There are currently two types of aortic prosthesis in clinical use.

CoreValve

The CoreValve prosthesis is a trileaflet porcine pericardial bioprosthesis mounted in a Nitinol stent with an overall length of 50mm and internal diameter of 21mm when fully expanded (Fig. 13.8). The stent has three distinct sections—a proximal portion which expands and excludes the native leaflets, a central portion constrained to avoid occlusion of the coronary ostia, and a distal portion which flares to fix the stent in the ascending aorta. Current generation valves can be delivered using an 18-French arterial sheath, reducing complications previously seen with the earlier 24-French system.

Arterial access may be femoral, subclavian, or axillary, usually with the patient intubated and sedated to facilitate transoesophageal monitoring. Initial balloon valvuloplasty during rapid ventricular pacing is followed by retrograde passage of the prosthesis across the valve. Deployment is undertaken using echocardiographic and fluoroscopic surveillance.

Edwards Sapien Valve

The Edwards Sapien prosthesis consists of a trileaflet equine pericardial bioprosthesis mounted within a short balloon expandable stent. The system is available in 23mm or 26mm diameter, requiring delivery through a 18 or 19-French system (Fig. 13.9). The valve can be delivered retrogradely via the femoral artery using the same principles as the Corevalve procedure or antegradely via puncture at the LV apex.

The retrograde approach utilizes a specialized delivery catheter to navigate the aortic arch and following balloon valvuloplasty the valve is deployed during rapid ventricular pacing; an antegrade approach via a short thoracotomy overlying the cardiac apex is an alternative. Following valvuloplasty a 24-French sheath is inserted and the prosthesis inserted over a wire under transoesophageal and fluoroscopic guidance (Fig. 13.7). Once the value is deployed the sheath is removed and previously placed pledgeted sutures tied to close the ventriculotomy.

This procedure requires unique collaboration between the cardiac surgeon and interventional cardiologist and is a viable alternative for patients who are unsuitable for conventional valve surgery in whom peripheral vascular access is not feasible.

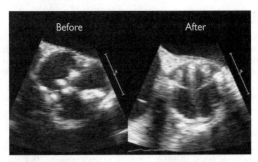

Fig. 13.7 Transoesophageal echocardiographic images before and after deployment of an Edwards Sapien prosthesis.

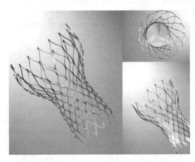

Fig. 13.8 Medtronic Corevalve device deployable via an 18 French delivery system. Reproduced from www.medtronic.com/core valve. © 2010 Medtronic, Inc. See also **Plate 26**.

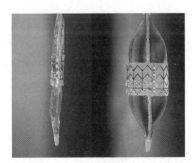

Fig. 13.9 The Edwards Sapien valve. See also **Plate 27**.
Taken from http://www.edwards.com/products/transcathetervalves/sapienhv.htm. Reproduced with permission from Edwards Lifesciences, Irvine California.

Pulmonary balloon valvuloplasty

Balloon valvuloplasty for isolated PS is a longstanding and highly effective treatment with excellent outcomes (Fig. 13.10). A degree of regurgitation is inevitable but rarely of clinical significance. The long term outcomes are similar to surgical intervention with low recurrence rates at 20 years.

Balloon dilation should be considered in:
- Symptomatic PS with a peak gradient >30mmHg
- Asymptomatic patients with peak gradient >40mmHg
- Critically unstable patients as a bridge to surgery
- Relief of obstruction in pregnancy (very rarely needed).

The procedure involves passage of a guidewire across the stenosed pulmonary valve followed by progressive balloon dilation. The aim is to stretch the pulmonary valve leaflets and allow elastic expansion of the annulus in order to relieve obstruction. Calcific PS is extremely rare.

Modest reductions in transvalvular gradients are usually seen. Long term outcomes are good, although repeated interventions may be required.

Not unexpectedly, the procedure carries a risk of significant complications including:
- Acute PR
- Cardiac tamponade
- Arrhythmia
- Pulmonary embolism and infarction
- Access site complications.

Contraindications

The presence of PR is a relative contraindication, since this will worsen as a result of the procedure. The balance of risks and benefits needs to be assessed in each individual patient.

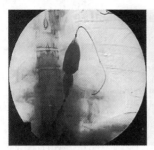 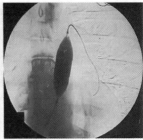

Fig. 13.10 Fluoroscopic image of a pulmonary balloon valvuloplasty. Reproduced with permission from Keane D., Jackson G. Percutaneous balloon pulmonary valvuloplasty. *NEJM*:331:846. Copyright 1994 Massachusetts Medical Society. All rights reserved.

Percutaneous pulmonary valve implantation

Acquired pulmonary valvular heart disease is rare and the percutaneous treatment of PR in adults is largely reserved for patients with corrected congenital lesions (typically patch augmentation of the RV outflow tract as part of corrective surgery for Fallot's tetralogy). Valved conduits placed between the RV and pulmonary artery may also develop calcific degeneration with resultant PS.

Implantation of the Melody valve (Medtronic) has been undertaken in hundreds of patients with repaired congenital disease worldwide with excellent results. The valve is a bovine jugular venous valve refined and sutured inside a balloon expandable stent delivered transvenously to the RV outflow tract (Fig. 13.11). Care must be taken to ensure anomalous coronary arteries are not compressed and that annular patch material has not become aneurysmal.

Tricuspid valvuloplasty

TS can also be treated percutaneously with balloon valvuloplasty in a manner similar to balloon mitral valvuloplasty. However, data are lacking on the long term outcome of this rarely performed procedure which should not be considered a definitive or durable treatment.

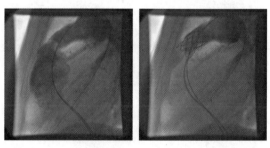

Fig. 13.11 Contrast angiography before and after deployment of a Melody valve within a degenerative valved conduit. The right hand panel demonstrates marked reduction in the degree of pulmonary regurgitation Reproduced from Coats, Bonhoeffer (2007) New percutaneous treatments for valve disease *Heart;* 93:639–644) with permission of BMJ Publishing Group Ltd.

Management during non-cardiac surgery

Introduction

Patients with valvular heart disease are at increased risk of morbidity and mortality during non-cardiac surgery. The ageing population and increasing numbers of surgical procedures in those aged >75 years mean that elderly patients with valvular heart disease are an increasingly frequent challenge.

The risk of non-cardiac surgery is dependent on the combination of patient specific factors and surgical procedural issues, including:
• Severity of valvular heart disease and underlying cardiac function
• Symptoms and functional status of the patient
• Nature of surgery and anaesthesia involved
• Risk of large volume loss or fluid shifts
• Length of procedure
• Comorbidities, including ischaemic heart disease.

The extent to which a patient is assessed and investigated is dictated largely by the nature and timing of surgery. In emergency cases there may only be time for a brief examination—however, identification of significant valvular heart disease will influence peri- and postoperative care, and a more complete evaluation can be undertaken afterwards. Non-urgent elective cases should be deferred until a thorough assessment is complete.

Assessment should include:
• History (including symptoms and comorbid disease)
• Estimation of functional status
• Physical examination
• 12 lead ECG
• Echocardiogram if valvular heart disease is suspected.

Frequently this will provide sufficient information to estimate the patient's risk during non-cardiac surgery and guide further management. In some patients additional non-invasive (e.g. dobutamine stress echocardiography) and invasive (e.g. left and right heart catheterization) investigations may be appropriate.

If significant valvular heart disease is identified, the risks of proceeding with surgery and the risks of delaying to allow optimal therapy +/− definitive intervention need to be compared. The proposed non-cardiac surgery can then be performed at a later date. Alternatively, in high risk cases, the absolute need for non-cardiac surgery should be re-addressed.

Estimating surgical risk

Although precise quantification is impossible in individual patients, non-cardiac surgical procedures can be identified as high, medium or low risk. Low risk procedures have a combined incidence of cardiac death or non-fatal myocardial infarction <1%, whereas this may exceed 5% in high risk procedures.

Emergency surgery in the elderly (>80 years) carries the highest risk. Vascular surgery is high risk due to the increased rates of coronary artery disease in this patient group.

Low risk	Medium risk	High risk
Endoscopic procedures	Carotid endarterectomy	Emergency surgery
Dermatological procedures	Head and neck surgery	Aortic surgery
Cataract surgery	Abdominal surgery*	Peripheral vascular surgery
Breast surgery	Thoracic surgery*	Prolonged procedure
Minor orthopaedic surgery (e.g. arthroscopy)	Major orthopaedic surgery (spine, hip)*	Expected significant blood loss
Minor urological surgery	Prostate surgery	Surgery in the elderly

*if uncomplicated

Estimating patient risk

Patient factors (age, comorbidities, current cardiovascular status, and degree of valvular heart disease) can also be classified into low, medium, and high risk:

Low risk	Medium risk	High risk
Advanced age	Mild stable angina	Recent myocardial infarction (<30 days)
Atrial fibrillation	Previous myocardial infarction	Unstable angina
Good functional capacity	Stable heart failure	Decompensated heart failure
Prior stroke	Diabetes mellitus	Major arrhythmia
Poor control of hypertension	Renal impairment	Severe valvular heart disease (eg VT)

An elderly patient with severe AS and decompensated heart failure is therefore an extremely high risk case.

Predicting risk before elective surgery is more feasible than in emergency situations. A range of risk scores have been developed, the most commonly used being the revised cardiac risk index which identifies six major risk factors:
- Ischaemic heart disease
- Planned high risk surgery
- Heart failure
- Stroke or transient ischaemic attack
- Diabetes mellitus treated with insulin
- Renal impairment.

Each factor is allocated a score of 1; the total score may then be used to estimate the risk of major cardiac complications:
- Score of 0 = 0.4%
- Score of 1 = 0.9%
- Score of 2 = 7%
- Score ≥3 = 11%.

Aortic stenosis

Major non-cardiac surgery

Severe AS is a major risk factor for perioperative morbidity and mortality during major non-cardiac surgery even in asymptomatic patients. If surgery cannot be deferred, then careful perioperative monitoring (often with invasive haemodynamic assessment) and appropriate anaesthetic support should be available.

Abrupt fall in preload, prolonged tachycardia (including atrial fibrillation) and decreasing systemic vascular resistance should all be avoided given the fixed obstruction to cardiac output. Peripheral vasoconstriction with phenylephrine can be used to treat intra-operative hypotension.

Elective aortic valve replacement (or balloon valvuloplasty in unsuitable cases) may be appropriate prior to major non-cardiac surgery, especially if the patient is symptomatic.

Other surgery

Low or medium risk surgery can be safely undertaken in patients with asymptomatic severe AS. Patients with symptoms should be considered for initial valve surgery unless emergency non-cardiac surgery is required.

Algorithm for severe aortic stenosis and non-cardiac surgery

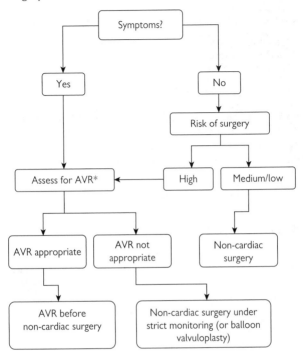

* AVR Aortic valve replacement

Mitral stenosis

Asymptomatic mitral stenosis

Non-cardiac surgery can be safely performed in patients with asymptomatic MS (even if severe) providing the pulmonary arterial systolic pressure is <50mmHg. Strict attention must be paid to:

• Avoidance of tachycardia
• Preservation of sinus rhythm
• Avoidance of fluid overload
• Anticoagulation requirements.

Asymptomatic patients with severe MS and significant pulmonary hypertension (pulmonary arterial systolic pressure >50mmHg) should be considered for intervention prior to major non-cardiac surgery.

Symptomatic mitral stenosis

Patients with symptomatic severe MS who require high risk non-cardiac surgery are at high risk of decompensation during physiological stress or arrhythmia. Initial valve intervention (percutaneous or surgical according to suitability) should be considered.

Aortic regurgitation

Asymptomatic aortic regurgitation

Patients with severe AR but no symptoms and preserved LV systolic function are at low risk for major cardiac events during non-cardiac surgery.

Symptomatic or decompensated aortic regurgitation

If LV function is preserved then optimization of medical therapy (including vasodilators and diuretics to ensure haemodynamic stability) prior to non-cardiac surgery is often sufficient.

If LV dysfunction (EF <50%) and other standard criteria for intervention are present (see 📖 p.148), then initial valve surgery should be considered. If this is not possible due to excessive risk then non-cardiac surgery should only be performed if absolutely necessary and with careful haemodynamic monitoring.

Mitral regurgitation

Asymptomatic mitral regurgitation

Asymptomatic patients with mild or moderate MR can safely undergo non-cardiac surgery at low risk without specific measures.

Asymptomatic patients with severe MR and preserved LV function (LVEF >60%) are also at low risk for major events during non-cardiac surgery.

Symptomatic or decompensated mitral regurgitation

Patients with either symptomatic severe MR or evidence of severe LV impairment (ejection fraction <30%) are at high risk of major cardiac events during non-cardiac surgery and need careful assessment and consideration of the optimal strategy:

- Optimize medical therapy (including vasodilators) and proceed with non-cardiac surgery

or

- Corrective valve surgery before proceeding with non-cardiac surgery.

Many factors will influence the optimal strategy, particularly the indication and urgency of the proposed non-cardiac surgery.

Pulmonary and tricuspid valve disease

Severe limiting disease of the pulmonary or tricuspid valve is much rarer, and experience during non-cardiac surgery is limited.

The principles of management remain:

- Stable asymptomatic patients can undergo non-cardiac surgery at low risk
- Patients with symptoms or evidence of marked cardiac decompensation require optimised medical therapy and consideration of definitive intervention (valve surgery) before non-cardiac surgery
- Patients requiring urgent non-cardiac surgery or patients unsuitable for definitive valve intervention require optimized medical therapy and close perioperative monitoring.

Prosthetic valves

The presence of a normally functioning prosthetic valve does not directly increase the risk of non-cardiac surgery. However, the need for anticoagulation in patients with mechanical prostheses can influence the risk of perioperative bleeding and subsequent complications.

Bridging anticoagulation

The optimal management of perioperative anticoagulation is dependent on patient and surgical factors, including:

• Risk of thrombosis relating to type and position of the prosthesis (see 📖 p.282)
• Type of surgery—bleeding risk and implications of haemorrhage
• Underlying risk of thrombosis—increased in surgery for malignancy or infection.

Surgery also affects the haemostatic pathways via multiple mechanisms; increased platelet activation, depression of fibrinolysis and effects of blood transfusion. Although difficult to quantify, the net effect is usually a pro-coagulant state with increased risk of valve thrombosis.

Low bleeding risk

For superficial procedures (e.g. dental work, skin biopsies) and other operations unlikely to cause major bleeding, the patient should be maintained on oral anticoagulation with the INR maintained at the lower end of the therapeutic range. Brief interruption of therapy for 1–3 days may be necessary to lower the INR but bridging heparin therapy is unnecessary if the INR remains in the therapeutic range.

If the procedure is uneventful then the usual dose of oral anticoagulation should be given on the day of the procedure and continued thereafter. Patients may require more frequent monitoring of the INR, particularly if post procedural antibiotics are given. Bleeding following dental extraction can be managed with oral tranexamic acid mouth wash.

Cardiac catheterization

Cardiac catheterization can be safely performed via the femoral artery if the INR is <2.0 particularly if a vascular closure device is employed. Access via the radial artery is safe with an INR <3.0. Pacemaker and defibrillator procedures can be safely performed if the INR is <3.0.

High bleeding risk

Many procedures cannot be performed safely whilst anticoagulation is maintained, either due to excessive bleeding risk or unacceptable potential complications of bleeding (e.g. following thyroid or neurosurgery). In such cases, oral anticoagulation is suspended several days before surgery and replaced with heparin once the INR falls below the therapeutic range for that patient.

Continuous infusion of unfractionated heparin dose adjusted to maintain a therapeutic APTT ratio is the preferred regime. The infusion is stopped before surgery (typically 6 hours) to allow the APTT ratio to normalize and restarted 6–12 hours following surgery once haemostasis is confirmed. Warfarin is re-introduced once bleeding risk is acceptable and heparin continued until the INR returns to the target range. Again, intensive INR monitoring is appropriate until the patient has fully recovered.

Low molecular weight heparin

Continuous intravenous infusion and the need for frequent APTT monitoring with unfractionated heparin prolong in-patient care and increase costs. Furthermore maintenance of the APTT within target range can be difficult. Weight-adjusted low molecular weight heparin has been studied in this setting and appears to be safe and equivalent to unfractionated heparin but is not currently licensed for this specific indication.

Doses require adjustment in renal impairment using the lowest dose possible to provide an anti-factor Xa level of 0.5–1.0IU/mL. Care must be taken in high risk patients such as those with older generation mitral prostheses (see 📖 p.282). Importantly, the effects of low molecular weight heparin last at least 12 hours and cannot be as easily or rapidly reversed.

Emergency non-cardiac surgery

This scenario should be managed in the same way as a patient with elevated INR and bleeding (see 📖 p.291).

The choice of reversing anticoagulation with vitamin K, fresh frozen plasma, or prothrombin complex concentrate depends on the urgency of surgery, potential bleeding risk, and INR level.

Following emergency surgery, the choice of subsequent anticoagulation will depend on the surgery performed and the postoperative bleeding risk. Unfractionated heparin should be reintroduced as soon as safely possible with close monitoring of the APTT ratio.

In some scenarios postoperative anticoagulation is not possible—e.g. following surgery for intra-cranial haemorrhage. Balancing the risk of anticoagulation against the risk of valve thrombosis requires early multidisciplinary team involvement.

Valvular heart disease in pregnancy

Introduction

Pregnancy places extra challenges on the cardiovascular system and can have significant implications for a patient with valvular heart disease, which fortunately complicates <1% of all pregnancies.

Close collaboration between the cardiologist, obstetrician, and patient is required at all stages, commencing ideally before pregnancy is even contemplated.

With appropriate management, most women with valvular heart disease can tolerate pregnancy and deliver a healthy baby. High-risk cases should be referred to centres with appropriate expertise and experience.

High risk valve lesions

The following scenarios carry high adverse event rates for the mother and foetus:

• Severe AS with or without symptoms
• Severe symptomatic AR, particularly if ejection fraction <40%
• Severe symptomatic MS, particularly if associated with severe pulmonary hypertension
• Severe symptomatic MR, particularly if ejection fraction <40%
• Severe symptomatic PS.

Haemodynamic changes of pregnancy

Marked changes occur in the cardiovascular system during pregnancy as a result of the uterine/placental circulation and hormonal effects. These include:

• 30–50% increase in cardiac output—due to increases in both heart rate (10–20bpm) and stroke volume, with resultant flow murmur
• Reduced systemic vascular resistance
• Reduced haematocrit.

These changes begin in the first trimester, plateau early in the second trimester, and increase further in the weeks before term until delivery.

Delivery

Delivery itself places further stresses on the cardiovascular system due to the physical challenges of labour and accompanying sympathetic drive:

• ↑ cardiac output
• ↑ heart rate
• ↑ blood pressure
• ↑ systemic vascular resistance.

Delivery of the placenta leads to an abrupt rise in both preload and afterload.

In the first 12–24 hours following delivery patients are at risk of heart failure as a consequence of increased venous return:

• Blood returning from the empty uterus
• Decreased caval compression
• Mobilisation of fluid from the lower limbs.

Normal clinical findings

The assessment of patients during pregnancy can be challenging, since there are many findings consistent with normal pregnancy:

- Fatigue
- Mild-moderate shortness of breath
- Palpitation, re-entrant supraventricular tachycardia
- Atrial and ventricular premature beats
- Raised jugular venous pressure
- Pedal oedema
- Sinus tachycardia
- Full volume, collapsing pulse
- Third heart sound
- Systolic flow murmur.

Clinical indicators of pathology

- Chest pain
- Severe dyspnoea
- Orthopnoea, paroxysmal nocturnal dyspnoea
- Sinus tachycardia >100/min at rest
- Atrial fibrillation/flutter
- Ventricular tachycardia
- Hypotension
- Pulmonary oedema
- Pleural effusion.

Murmurs in pregnancy

Systolic flow murmurs are common in pregnancy due to increased cardiac output. An 'innocent' murmur should be soft, systolic, and usually best heard at the left sternal edge without any other signs of valvular heart disease. Murmurs which are loud (≥3/6), diastolic, or associated with radiation or a thrill are not 'normal' and suggest a significant lesion requiring assessment with echocardiography.

Who to refer for echocardiography

- Patients with a significant murmur (see above)
- Anyone with other signs of valvular heart disease
- Patients with significant breathlessness.

General management

Assessment of risk

The assessment of a patient with valvular heart disease who is (or is intending to become) pregnant should focus on:
- History—baseline exercise tolerance
- Examination—evidence of decompensation, change in murmur
- Echocardiography—assessment of valve function and pulmonary arterial pressure.

The risk of complications during pregnancy can be assessed according to the type and severity of valvular heart disease.

Patients with mild valvular heart disease can be reviewed monthly during the antenatal period. Those with more severe disease may need review every two weeks until 30 weeks, and every week thereafter.

Management

Patients with high risk valve lesions require expert management. Advice from a cardiologist experienced in managing valvular heart disease in pregnancy should be sought. All require close monitoring and some may require intervention during (or immediately following) pregnancy—either balloon valvuloplasty or valve replacement.

Minimizing cardiovascular demand

Bed-rest and oxygen are useful to minimize the cardiovascular demands of pregnancy in symptomatic patients. Avoidance of pain, anxiety, infection, and dehydration are also important.

Drugs

Diuretics, β-blockers, hydralazine, and digoxin can be safely used in pregnancy if required. ACE inhibitors, amiodarone, and nitroprusside are teratogenic and should be avoided.

Labour

- Planning of appropriate haemodynamic monitoring and expert support to mother and foetus are of utmost importance in ensuring a safe delivery
- Caesarean section results in greater haemodynamic change and blood loss than vaginal delivery and should only be used for foetal indications. The physical exertion of normal vaginal delivery should be minimized by use of forceps or suction devices
- Antibiotic prophylaxis (to prevent IE) is no longer required.

Lesion	Low risk	High risk
All	NYHA class I	Symptoms on modest exertion (NYHA class ˜II)
All	LV ejection fraction >55%	LV ejection fraction <40%
All	Normal pulmonary arterial pressure	Pulmonary hypertension (>50% systemic pressure)
AS	Asymptomatic mild to moderate AS	Severe AS
AR	Asymptomatic mild–moderate AR, normal LV size and function	Symptomatic severe AR
MS	Asymptomatic mild–moderate MS	Severe or symptomatic MS
MR	Asymptomatic mild–moderate MR, normal LV size and function	Symptomatic severe MR

General principles of cardiac management

Avoid medication if possible. If necessary, use the fewest agents in the smallest possible doses

BUT

- Do not deny appropriate management simply because of pregnancy
- In particular, do not withhold imaging involving radiation if the mother has a possible life-threatening condition (e.g. pulmonary embolism).

▶ REMEMBER: if the mother is compromised, so is the foetus.

▶ Obtain EARLY advice from:

- 'High-risk' obstetrician
- Cardiologist with expertise in pregnancy.

Drugs for valvular heart disease in pregnancy

Drug	Indication	Potential effect to the foetus
ACE inhibitor	Contraindicated	Urogenital defects, growth retardation and foetal death
Adenosine	Termination of arrhythmia	No adverse effects
Amiodarone	Treatment of arrhythmias in very high risk patients	Hypothyroidism and premature delivery
β blocker	Control of heart rate and blood pressure	Reduced heart rate and birth weight
Digoxin	Control of heart rate	No adverse effects
Furosemide	Treatment of fluid overload	Increased urinary sodium and potassium loss
Heparin	Anticoagulation	Foetal haemorrhage
Hydralazine	Vasodilation	No adverse effects
Methyldopa	Treatment of hypertension	No adverse effects
Nitrates	Vasodilation	Reduced heart rate
Nitroprusside	Treatment of hypertension	Potential cyanide toxicity
Warfarin	Anticoagulation of mechanical prosthesis	Developmental (craniofacial) abnormalities if used between weeks 6–12 of pregnancy*, foetal haemorrhage

*minimal risk if daily dose <5mg.

Aortic stenosis in pregnancy

Most cases of AS associated with pregnancy in developed nations relate to a bicuspid valve. Rheumatic AS is still common in developing nations.

Mild to moderate aortic stenosis

Rarely leads to problems if LV function is normal and can be managed conservatively with intermittent monitoring.

Severe aortic stenosis

Even severe AS is usually well tolerated in pregnancy if:
- Asymptomatic
- Peak pressure drop <80mmHg (mean <50mmHg) before pregnancy
- Normal LV function
- No exercise induced symptoms at 100% of predicted target heart rate for age.

Asymptomatic severe AS requires close monitoring during pregnancy for symptoms, signs of heart failure or LV dysfunction.

Monitoring

The aortic valve gradient climbs steadily as cardiac output increases during pregnancy. Failure to do so suggests the possibility of associated LV impairment.

Development of symptoms

If severe symptomatic AS is detected during pregnancy (or symptoms develop in a previously asymptomatic patient), bed rest, diuretics, and β blockade may be helpful. If pregnancy is sufficiently advanced, delivery followed by standard treatment of AS is preferred. Balloon valvuloplasty may be required as a holding measure with definitive intervention (valve replacement) following delivery. Vaginal delivery is preferable—if Caesarean section is needed then this should be performed under general anaesthesia.

Valve replacement during pregnancy carries a maternal mortality risk of 6% and a foetal mortality risk of 30%, but may still be necessary in severe cases (e.g. critical pulmonary oedema or recurrent syncope). In later stages of pregnancy, delivery by Caesarean section followed by immediate valve replacement is often recommended.

If severe AS is identified before pregnancy then conception should be delayed to allow valve replacement. Careful consideration should be given to the choice of prosthesis and required anticoagulation regime.

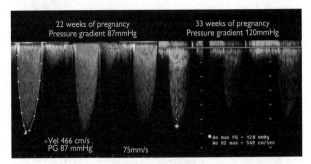

Fig. 15.1 Changes in aortic valve gradient with pregnancy. This patient required emergency aortic valve replacement at 36 weeks due to the development of refractory heart failure.

Mitral stenosis in pregnancy

Rheumatic MS is the most frequent valve disorder encountered during pregnancy and often remains asymptomatic until unmasked by pregnancy. Mild to moderate MS is usually well tolerated, but problems may arise if valve area is <1.5cm^2 even if the patient was asymptomatic before conception.

Patients with known severe MS who are contemplating pregnancy should be assessed for balloon mitral valvuloplasty and undergo this procedure if suitable. If there are contraindications to percutaneous intervention then the risks of pregnancy with MS have to be balanced against the risks of pregnancy with a prosthetic valve.

Patients are susceptible to the increased circulating volume and heart rate during the second trimester of pregnancy. Both increase left atrial pressure, potentially causing decompensation, heart failure, and acute pulmonary oedema. This can be abrupt, particularly at the onset of atrial fibrillation. Typically symptoms increase by at least one functional class during pregnancy. The average gestational age at which pulmonary oedema develops is 30 weeks and 20% of these arise due to the onset of an atrial tachyarrhythmia.

Management

Medical therapy aims to reduce heart rate and left atrial pressure, and includes bed rest, oxygen, diuretics, and β blockers. Any concomitant infection should be promptly treated with appropriate antibiotics.

β-blockers are safe in pregnancy – metoprolol is frequently preferred since it is more cardiospecific. Older agents, such as atenolol, have been associated with intra-uterine growth retardation. Digoxin and verapamil are suitable alternatives if β-blockers are contraindicated e.g. asthma.

Salt restriction and careful diuretic therapy can help reduce circulating volume and left atrial pressure. Care is required to avoid hypotension and placental hypoperfusion.

Balloon mitral valvuloplasty can be performed during pregnancy with minimal risk to the mother and foetus (transoesophogeal echocardiographic monitoring can minimise the radiation requirement) and should be considered if:

• Severe symptoms despite medical therapy
• Pulmonary arterial pressure > 50mmHg.

Additional management points

- If the degree of MR prevents balloon mitral valvuloplasty, mitral valve surgery should be considered in patients with severe MS refractory to medical therapy. Surgical success has been reported in pregnancy but the risk of foetal mortality is around 30% and maternal mortality as high as 10%.
- Anticoagulation with heparin should be considered if there is associated atrial fibrillation or marked left atrial dilation.
- Caesarean section is only indicated for obstetric reasons. Vaginal delivery is safe, even in severe MS, if measures are taken to shorten the second stage of labour (epidural anaesthesia, forceps or suction extraction). Careful haemodynamic monitoring is recommended and should continue for at least 24 hours after delivery.

Aortic regurgitation in pregnancy

Pregnancy is well tolerated by women with chronic AR with normal LV function and rarely requires intervention. Decreased systemic vascular resistance and increasing heart rate reduce both the duration of diastole and the pressure differential between the aorta and LV, reducing the degree of AR.

Symptomatic patients with AR and LV dilation require treatment with vasodilators, salt restriction, and diuretics. ACE inhibitors are contraindicated in pregnancy but hydralazine/nitrate combinations provide a good alternative. Haemodynamic monitoring and expert cardiology input are required during labour—valve replacement should always be deferred until the post-partum period if at all possible, as the risk of foetal loss is high.

AR associated with Marfan's syndrome and an aortic root diameter >40mm presents a high risk of aortic complications (particularly dissection). These patients need expert management with careful echocardiographic follow up and early surgery may be required.

Mitral regurgitation in pregnancy

Chronic MR with normal LV function is usually well tolerated as the reduced afterload of pregnancy is beneficial.

During labour, the increase in both preload and afterload following placental delivery can cause pulmonary oedema. Diuretics and vasodilation may be useful in the first 24–48 hours following delivery.

Mitral valve surgery is virtually never needed for MR during pregnancy and should only be considered in patients with severe refractory symptoms as rates of foetal mortality are high.

Acute severe MR due to valve disruption (complicating myocardial infarction or IE) is rare but presents a surgical emergency requiring immediate treatment to achieve haemodynamic stability (often with an intra-aortic balloon pump) before surgical intervention.

Pulmonary stenosis in pregnancy

Isolated PS may relate to congenital abnormality of the valve or degeneration of a homograft implanted as part of a Ross procedure.

- Severe PS is usually well tolerated during pregnancy unless there is significant RV failure.
- Balloon valvuloplasty is the treatment of choice if there is symptomatic deterioration.
- Newer stent-valve devices can be useful, particularly if there is significant PR. However, the requirement for short term anti-platelet therapy may present problems during pregnancy and these procedures are usually deferred to the post partum period if possible.

Tricuspid regurgitation in pregnancy

Chronic TR is well tolerated in pregnancy, even if severe, providing that RV function is not severely impaired. Medical therapy focussing on maintenance of sinus rhythm, diuretics and salt restriction is usually sufficient.

Prosthetic valves in pregnancy

The management of prosthetic valves during pregnancy requires planned changes in anticoagulation and careful multidisciplinary care (see 📖 p.302).

Infective endocarditis

Introduction

IE is a potentially lethal disease despite advances in diagnosis, medical, and surgical therapy. Although overall incidence has not changed significantly, the clinical profile has—more cases now affect the elderly and those with prosthetic valves and other cardiac devices.

Clinical presentation is diverse and often vague, making diagnosis a challenge. A high index of suspicion and low threshold for investigation are necessary in patients at high risk of IE to ensure the disease is not missed at an early (and potentially treatable) stage.

Optimal management can only be achieved with the input of a wide variety of specialists, including cardiologists, microbiologists, cardiac surgeons, and infectious disease specialists. Complications (Fig. 16.1) may warrant the involvement of neurologists and neurosurgeons, vascular and general surgeons, pathologists, and imaging specialists. Multidisciplinary discussions and planning are particularly important in complex cases.

Epidemiology

As in other forms of valvular heart disease, the decline of rheumatic fever has changed the profile of this condition. Young patients with IE complicating rheumatic valvular heart disease are now rare, whereas IE secondary to health care-related infection or intravenous drug abuse is increasingly common.

These changes have been accompanied by increasing frequency of staphylococcal infection, which now exceeds streptococcal infection in developed nations. Elderly patients are also more common, reflecting their increased prevalence of degenerative valvular heart disease and rising rates of invasive medical procedures in this group.

Overall incidence of IE varies between 1.4–11.6 episodes per 100,000 person-years with highest rates seen in patients >70 years of age. Men are afflicted three times more frequently than women.

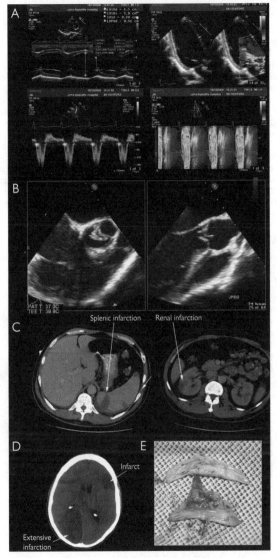

Fig. 16.1 Examples of the complications of infective endocarditis. See also **Plate 28** (A) severe aortic regurgitation and LV dilation; (B) perforated bicuspid aortic valve; (C) splenic and renal infarction; (D) cerebral infarction; (E) perforated bicuspid aortic valve with regurgitation at surgery. All these complications were present in the same patient who had streptococcal endocarditis of a bicuspid aortic valve.

Pathophysiology

Bacteraemia, usually related to day to day activities (e.g. mastication, tooth brushing) or invasive dental or medical procedures, is required to cause IE, though why only a few bacteraemias cause problems is unclear. A predisposition to infection (eg valve lesions/damage) may provide part of the reason, and abnormalities of the valvular endothelium allow platelet aggregation and fibrin deposition with subsequent bacterial adherence, multiplication and endothelial invasion.

Vegetations (Fig. 16.2 & 16.3), the hallmark of IE, consist of fibrin, platelets, leucocytes and bacterial clusters. Histiocytes and monocytes are found deep within, whereas the surface usually consists of fibrin and leucocytes. Vegetations are avascular and bacteria may thrive despite high plasma antibiotic concentrations, explaining (in part) the need for prolonged antimicrobial therapy.

Risk factors

In many patients with IE, no overt risk factor can be identified. Assessment of a patient's potential risk of acquiring IE is important to guide appropriate education and use of antibiotic prophylaxis.

High risk features (see 📖 p.389)
• Prosthetic valve—mechanical or biological
• Previous IE—even if cure achieved
• Cyanotic congenital heart disease
• Patent ductus arteriosus
• Left to right intra-cardiac shunt (e.g. ventricular septal defect)
• Significant native valvular heart disease.

Other clinical factors which increase the risk of acquiring IE and an adverse outcome of the condition include:
• Intravenous drug use
• Severe dental disease
• Carcinoma of the colon (associated with *Streptococcus bovis*)
• Diabetes mellitus
• Immunosupression
• Renal failure
• Indwelling central venous catheter
• Pregnancy
• Arterio-venous fistulae.

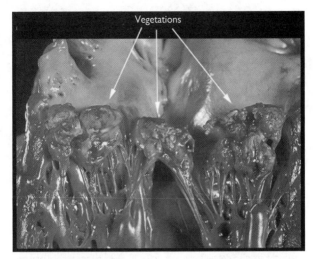

Fig. 16.2 Extensive vegetations on both leaflets of the mitral valve. Reproduced from the Public Health Image Library (PHIL) (⊗ http://phil.cdc.gov/PHIL_Images/02122002/00007/PHIL_851_lores.jpg)

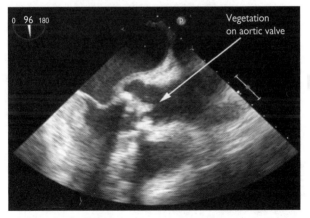

Fig. 16.3 Transoesophageal echocardiogram demonstrating a large mass of vegetations on the aortic valve.

Classification

A wide variety of cardiac, extra-cardiac, and microbiological factors may combine in IE leading to a very broad range of clinical scenarios, each with different treatment regimes and likely outcomes. Classification is based on the following factors:

• Native valve or prosthetic valve
• Left or right sided valve
• Device-related IE (pacemaker lead, catheter)
• Community acquired or healthcare associated infection
• Active or treated
• Relapse or re-infection
• Culture positive or negative.

Prosthetic valve infection can be further divided into early (<1 year of surgery) or late infection (>1 year since surgery).

Healthcare associated infection can be divided into nosocomial (acquired following >48 hours in hospital) or non-nosocomial (healthcare contact outside hospital, e.g. dialysis treatment, long term care facility).

Active IE implies clinical features of ongoing infection (persistent fever, persistently positive blood cultures, and active inflammation at surgery or histopathological evidence of active infection). Patients receiving antibiotic treatment are also defined as having active IE, even in the absence of these features.

Relapse is defined as re-infection with the same microorganism <6 months since the previous episode.

Re-infection implies a different microorganism or the same micro-organism >6 months since the previous episode.

Clinical signs

The constellation of clinical signs depends on the duration of infection and the presence or absence of cardiac and extra-cardiac complications. The patient should be carefully assessed with the following in mind:

Portal of infection
• Dental hygiene and periodontal disease
• Skin—particularly cannula sites or evidence of intravenous drug use
• Central venous or urinary catheters.

Evidence of infection
• Temperature
• Weight loss
• Confusion or encephalopathy
• Joint collections or abscesses
• Lymphadenopathy
• Clubbing
• Splenomegaly.

Cardiac involvement
- Murmur
- Signs of valvular regurgitation
- Signs of cardiac enlargement
- Signs of heart failure
- Heart rhythm (atrial fibrillation, heart block)
- Pericardial involvement (rub, effusion).

Haemodynamic status
- Heart rate and blood pressure
- Oxygenation and respiratory rate
- Peripheral perfusion, mental state and urine output
- Venous pressure
- Evidence of pulmonary oedema or infection.

Extra-cardiac involvement and immune mediated phenomena
- Neurological examination—cerebral/cerebellar infarcts or abscess
- Fundoscopy for Roth spots—retinal haemorrhages
- Conjunctivae and nail beds for splinter haemorrhages (Fig. 16.4)
- Hands and feet for Janeway lesions—flat non-tender red spots
- Fingers for Osler's nodes—tender pea sized nodules on finger pulps
- Arthritis or arthralgia
- Petechiae or bleeding.

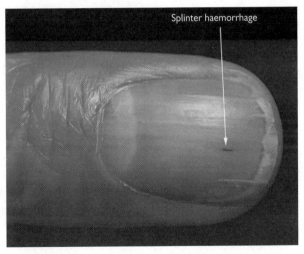

Splinter haemorrhage

Fig. 16.4 Splinter haemorrhage – thought to result from embolic occlusion of linear capillaries in the nail bed.

Clinical presentation

The spectrum of IE ranges from a sub-acute low grade illness to a fulminant acute disease associated with septicaemia, valve destruction, and cardiogenic shock. Clinical features depend on the interaction of potential cardiac, extra-cardiac and immune mediated effects:

Cardiac manifestations

These depend on the site of the lesion, underlying valvular heart disease, and baseline cardiac function (including coronary artery disease):

- New or changing murmur
- Heart failure
- Atrioventricular block
- Pericarditis
- Coronary ischaemia/infarction.

Extra-cardiac manifestations

These largely relate to the embolic potential of vegetations:

- Stroke/transient cerebral ischaemia
- Renal, splenic and hepatic emboli
- Joint collections/abscess
- Pulmonary abscess (septic emboli)
- Back pain—may be discitis
- Renal impairment—frequently multifactorial.

Immune mediated effects

These relate to vasculitic effects of the bacteraemia/septicaemia and the hosts immune response.

- Petechiae
- Splinter haemorrhages
- Janeway lesions and Osler's nodes
- Roth spots (retinal haemorrhages)
- Haematuria
- Glomerulonephritis
- Arthralgia/arthritis
- Encephalopathy.

Clinical features

The majority of patients with IE develop fever associated with systemic symptoms of malaise, reduced appetite, and weight loss. Night sweats are common and rigors may accompany episodes of bacteraemia. These features may be absent in the elderly and immunosuppressed.

A murmur is present in around 75% of cases and classical signs, e.g. Osler's nodes and Janeway lesions, are now rare as the majority of cases are more acute, with little time for immune-mediated features to appear. Clubbing, splenomegaly, lymphadenopathy, and non-specific anaemia are seen in chronic low grade infection (most usually related to streptococcal infection). Peripheral emboli are most common in the brain, may complicate up to one-third of cases, and are often the presenting feature. Systematic surveillance (e.g. by cerebral and abdominal CT scanning) may demonstrate an even higher frequency of clinically silent embolic complications.

These diverse manifestations mean that patients with IE frequently present to non-cardiac specialities, including haematology, rheumatology, neurology, infectious diseases, and vascular surgery. Constant awareness of the condition, particularly in high risk groups, is essential to ensure that the diagnosis is not overlooked and that appropriate investigations and treatment are instigated.

Diagnosis

Diagnosis requires an amalgamation of clinical, microbiological, and echocardiographic data. The modified Duke criteria (see 📖 p.358) are useful and have an overall accuracy of 80%, but do not replace clinical judgment and individual case assessment.

Blood cultures

Blood cultures are vital in the diagnosis of IE and must never be over-looked—multiple samples should be taken before antibiotic therapy is administered. Even in acute severe IE there is time for three separate sets to be obtained over one hour whilst the patient's condition is stabilized.

In stable subacute cases, 48 hours can be spent obtaining a series of care-fully sampled cultures to allow appropriately directed antibiotic therapy from the outset.

- Cultures must be taken from a peripheral vein using sterile technique to avoid contamination.
- Multiple sets (ideally >1 hour apart) are required from multiple sites.
- There is no need to coincide cultures with spikes of fever—bacteraemia in IE is virtually constant.
- Aim for at least 10ml in each aerobic and anaerobic sample to increase rates of detection (aerobic first, since anaerobes are rare).
- Provide the laboratory with detailed information on previous antibiotic use.
- Culture may be taken from an indwelling venous catheter in addition to (but NOT instead of) peripheral venous culture.
- Areas of cutaneous inflammation or infection should be swabbed and cultured separately.

Echocardiography

Imaging with both transthoracic and transoesophogeal echocardiography (TTE/TOE) is important in the diagnosis and assessment of IE
- The pre-test probability of IE is important for correct interpretation
- TTE has a sensitivity of only 50–60%: as many as half of the cases may be missed
- A 'negative' TTE (or TOE) does NOT exclude IE unless the clinical likelihood is low—follow up imaging may be required if suspicion is high
- False positives may arise if minor valve abnormalities are misinterpreted as vegetations—again the clinical scenario is crucial
- TOE has a sensitivity of ~ 95% but is invasive, more expensive and carries small risks.

In most patients, it is reasonable to perform an initial TTE. In those with a prosthetic valve and high clinical suspicion of IE (e.g. fever, positive blood cultures, and valve dysfunction) proceeding directly to TOE is appropriate. Virtually all patients with *confirmed* IE should undergo TOE to define valve anatomy and detect complications.

Additional investigations:

- Full blood count—anaemia, leucocytosis, thrombocytopenia
- Coagulation—coagulopathy, disseminated intravascular coagulation
- U & E—renal impairment, uraemia, hyperkalaemia
- Liver function—derangement may be multifactorial
- C-reactive protein—may be useful for monitoring progress
- Erythrocyte sedimentation rate—acute phase reactant.

Indications for echocardiography in suspected infective endocarditis

When clinical suspicion is high:
- New valve lesion (usually regurgitant murmur)
- Embolic events of unknown origin
- Sepsis (i.e. bacteraemia plus systemic features) of unknown origin
- Haematuria, glomerulonephritis and suspected renal infarction
- Fever *plus*:
  - +ve blood cultures with organisms typical of IE
  - High predisposition for IE e.g. prosthetic valve
  - First manifestation of heart failure
  - Newly-developed conduction disturbance or ventricular arrhythmia
  - Typical immunological manifestations of IE
  - Multifocal/rapidly changing pulmonary infiltrates
  - Peripheral abscesses of unknown origin (e.g. renal, splenic, and spinal)
  - Predisposition plus recent diagnostic/therapeutic intervention known to result in significant bacteraemia.

NB: a fever without other evidence for IE is not an indication for echocardiography.

Indications for transoesophageal echocardiography (see p.590)

- Positive TTE – assess valve lesion in more detail and exclude high risk complications, e.g. abscess formation
- Non-diagnostic TTE with high clinical suspicion of IE
- Prosthetic valve IE – TTE is rarely diagnostic
- Technically difficult TTE with sufficient clinical suspicion of IE
- Initially negative TOE but high clinical suspicion of IE – repeat TOE after 7–10 days
- Confirmed IE with evidence of progression or new complication, e.g. new heart block or embolic event

Characteristics of vegetations

Vegetations have a number of typical features which facilitate echocardiographic identification:

- Texture similar to myocardium—(mid grey) bright lesions are more likely to be calcium
- 'Upstream' of valve—atrial side of atrioventricular valves and ventricular side of ventriculo-arterial valves
- Oscillatory motion and 'upstream' prolapse
- Location alongside the path of any regurgitant jet
- Attached to prosthetic material
- Lobulated shape—thread like structures are unlikely to be vegetations
- Supportive findings—a mass is more likely to be a vegetation in the presence of significant valvular regurgitation, abscess formation, fistulae, or prosthetic dehiscence.

The size and mobility of the vegetation are associated with embolic risk (Fig. 16.5 and Fig. 16.6).

Size

- Very small   <2mm
- Small   2–5mm
- Medium   5–10mm
- Large   >10mm

Mobility

- Absent—fixed vegetation with no independent motion
- Low—fixed base but mobile free edge
- Moderate—pedunculated vegetation which remains in same cardiac chamber throughout cardiac cycle
- Severe—pedunculated vegetation which crosses the valve leaflets during cardiac cycle.

Electrocardiogram

A baseline ECG may demonstrate arrhythmias, heart block (associated with perivalvular complications), myocardial ischaemia, or infarction (associated with coronary embolism).

Chest X-ray

Pulmonary oedema may complicate haemodynamic decompensation. Pulmonary infiltration, abscess, or infarction may be seen in right sided IE.

Urinalysis

Microscopic haematuria and proteinuria are associated with immune-mediated glomerulonephritis.

Mechanism of valve dysfunction

Valve destruction by IE leads to regurgitation, but the exact mechanism can vary. This should be clarified at the time of imaging to guide the need for intervention and choice of surgical procedure.

- Leaflet perforation.
- Leaflet destruction with resultant flail leaflet.
- Obstruction of leaflet co-aptation by large vegetation.
- Paravalvular regurgitation via abscess cavity.
- Prosthetic valve dehiscence.

Perivalvular complications

IE frequently involves paravalvular tissues resulting in formation of an abscess, pseudoaneurysm or fistula. Identification is vital since these complications are associated with increased mortality and need for surgery.

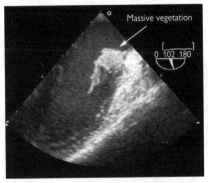

Fig. 16.5 Transoesophageal echocardiogram demonstrating an enormous vegetation on the atrial aspect of the posterior mitral valve leaflet with prolapse into the left ventricle.

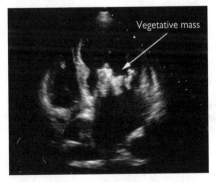

Fig. 16.6 Transthoracic echocardiogram demonstrating a huge vegetative mass encasing the entire mitral valve. This patient initially presented with non-specific symptoms and was mistakenly treated with steroids.

Duke criteria

The modified Duke criteria classify clinical, microbiological, and echocardiographic factors:

Definite IE
- 2 major criteria
- 1 major and 3 minor criteria
- 5 minor criteria.

Possible IE
- 1 major and 1 minor criteria
- 3 minor criteria.

Major criteria
- **Positive blood culture**
  - Microorganism typical of IE from two separate cultures
  - Persistently positive cultures with microorganism typical of IE
  - Single positive culture for *Coxiella burnetii* (or IgG titre >1:800).
- **Evidence of endocardial involvement**
  - Vegetation
  - Abscess
  - Prosthetic valve dehiscence
  - New valvular regurgitation.

Minor criteria
- **Predisposing condition:**
  - Structurally abnormal valve or prosthetic valve
  - Intravenous drug use.
- **Fever:**
  - Temperature > 38°C.
- **Vascular phenomena:**
  - Arterial emboli
  - Septic pulmonary infarction
  - Mycotic aneurysm
  - Intra-cranial haemorrhage
  - Conjunctival haemorrhage
  - Janeway lesions.
- **Immune mediated phenomena:**
  - Glomerulonephritis
  - Osler's nodes
  - Roth spots
  - Rheumatoid factor.
- **Microbiological evidence**:
  - Positive culture but microorganism not typical of IE
  - Serological evidence of infection with organism typical of IE.

Differential diagnosis

Incorrect diagnosis of IE occurs occasionally and usually relates to misinterpretation of echocardiographic or microbiological findings.

Alternative causes of a mobile echocardiographic mass

- Calcified valve lesions
- Lambl's excrescences (fibro-elastic protrusion on the aortic valve)
- Ruptured chordae or prolapsed valve leaflet
- Marantic vegetations (associated with advanced malignancy)
- Libman-Sacks endocarditis (associated with systemic lupus erythematosus)
- Nonbacterial thrombotic endocarditis
- Fibroelastoma
- Nodule of Arantius (thickened tip of aortic valve leaflet)
- Healed vegetation.

Vegetations usually regress following successful treatment of IE. Persistence can cause considerable diagnostic confusion unless imaging has been undertaken in the convalescent period.

Microbiology

Terminology describing the variety of pathogens that can cause IE is confusing for the non-specialist. Over 95% of cases are due to bacteria, and the majority of these are staphylococci or streptococci. Rarer causes include unusual bacteria and fungi.

Bacteria can be crudely divided according to cell wall properties into Gram-positive and Gram-negative species. Further subdivisions include the ability to promote coagulation (coagulase-positive, usually applied to staphylococci) and haemolysis (partial [alpha] or complete [β] haemolytic, usually applied to streptococci).

Gram positive bacteria

Many bacteria are Gram-positive but only the spherical cocci commonly cause IE. *Listeria Monocytogenes* is a Gram-positive bacillus and a rare cause of IE.

Gram negative bacteria

The HACEK group of organisms are Gram-negative and a frequent cause of IE. Additional pathogens include *Escherichia coli*, a common cause of gastrointestinal and urinary tract infections, and *Pseudomonas Aeruginosa*, which more commonly causes respiratory or urinary tract infections. IE may also be rarely caused by rickettsial pathogens, including *Coxiella burnetii* and *Bartonella* species.

Interpretation of positive blood culture

Not all microorganisms have the ability to invade endothelium and cause IE. Furthermore, a positive blood culture is more likely to reflect IE if there is no alternative source for the bacteraemia.

Typical organisms include:
• *Staphylococcus Aureus*
• *Streptococcus Viridans*
• *Streptococcus Bovis*
• *Enterococci*
• HACEK group.

The significance of a positive blood culture depends on the organism and its frequency of detection—for example, *Streptococcus Viridans* appearing in two cultures >12 hours apart is highly suggestive of IE, whereas *Corynebacterium* from 1 of 6 cultures is more likely to be a contaminant.

Gram Positive pathogens

Genus	Species	Classification	Source	Comment
Staphylococcus	aureus	Coagulase positive	Skin and nasal flora	Common
	epidermidis	Coagulase negative	Skin flora	Common in prosthetic valve endocarditis
Streptococcus	viridans Group*	Alpha haemolytic	Normal flora	Common
	pneumoniae	Alpha haemolytic	Respiratory flora	Rare
	pyogenes	β haemolytic group A	Infrequent skin flora	Causes rheumatic fever
	algactiae	β haemolytic group B	Urogenital flora	Rare—destructive disease
	bovis	Non haemolytic group D	Flora of ruminants	Associated with colonic disease
	canis	β haemolytic group G	Flora of dogs	Rare
Enterococcus	faecalis	Non haemolytic	Enter via urinary or gastrointestinal tract	Increasing cause of nosocomial infections
Listeria	mono-cytogenes	N/A	Soil, water and food	Rare with a high mortality

* mitis, mutans, oralis, sanguinis, gordonii, salivarius, lugdinensis, milleri

Gram negative pathogens

The HACEK group consists of the following organisms:

Genus	Species	Comment
Haemophilus	aphrophilus	More likely to involve mitral valve
	parainfluenzae	Increasing in frequency
Actinobacillus	actinomycete	High embolic risk
Cardiobacterium	hominis	Mouth and upper airway flora
Eikenella	corrodens	Associated with intravenous drug use—contamination from mouth flora
Kingella	kingae	Rapid progression typical

Additional gram negative pathogens include:

Genus	Species	Comment
Escherichia	coli	Rare—usually involves prosthetic valves
Pseudomonas	aeruginosa	Usually acute—high mortality without surgery

Other pathogens causing infective endocarditis

Genus	Species	Comment
Fungi	Candida	Associated with indwelling catheters
	Aspergillus	Can occur in postoperative patients
Bartonella	quintata	Transmitted by louse—suspect in homeless patients
	henslae	Causes cat scratch disease
Brucella	N/A	From unpasteurized milk—rare cause of IE
Coxiella	burnetii	Contact with cattle—long latent period

Complications

Potential complications of IE are many and varied:
- Heart failure—the most common indication for surgery, usually caused by severe valvular regurgitation (Fig. 16.7)
- Abscess formation—associated with high mortality
- Fistulae
- Stroke—cerebral or cerebellar embolism (Fig. 16.8)
- Ischaemic digits or limbs—peripheral embolism
- Myocardial infarction—coronary embolism
- Meningoencephalitis—may cause seizures
- Ruptured mycotic aneurysm
- Cerebral abscess
- Splenic abscess or infarction
- Renal infarction
- Osteomyelitis
- Vertebral abscess and discitis
- Mediastinitis—can also occur postoperatively.

Additional complications can relate to treatment:
- Ototoxicity from aminoglycoside therapy
- Nephrotoxicity from antimicrobial therapy (especially aminoglycoside)
- Drug-induced fever—often related to high dose antibiotic therapy
- Allergic reactions
- Nosocomial infections—usually related to venous or urinary catheters.

Natural history and prognosis

The overall mortality of IE remains as high as 30% at one year, with an in-hospital mortality of 20%. Up to 50% of patients require valve surgery which may be undertaken in the acute setting or convalescent phase.

Features associated with adverse outcome include:
- *Staphylococcus Aureus* infection
- Heart failure
- Perivalvular complications (abscess/fistula)
- Prosthetic valve infection
- Persistent bacteraemia
- Diabetes mellitus
- Large vegetation size
- Fungal infection
- Poor ventricular function.

These factors are cumulative—a patient with heart failure and perivalvular abscess due to *Staphylococcus Aureus* infection has a predicted one month mortality of 75%.

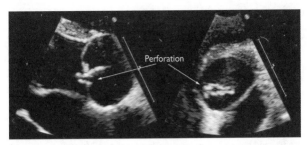

Fig. 16.7 Perforation of a bicuspid aortic valve due to infective endocarditis with severe aortic regurgitation.

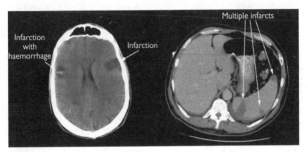

Fig. 16.8 Computed tomography imaging—the left hand panel demonstrates a cerebral infarct and the right hand panel a splenic infarction.

General management

Following diagnosis, patients with IE require prolonged treatment, close surveillance, frequent reassessment, and possible cardiac surgery. Correctly tailored antimicrobial therapy is the mainstay, but consideration should also be given to:

Venous access

Patients require frequent intravenous drug administration and venepuncture, both of which can become painful and distressing. Early use of long-term venous access, e.g. Hickman line or peripherally inserted central venous catheter (PICC), is recommended. These lines require meticulous sterility and should be regularly checked for signs of infection.

Nutrition

Patients with IE are usually catabolic and easily lose weight and muscle bulk. Appropriate nutritional assessment and advice should be provided and inpatients should remain mobile and active if feasible.

Thromboembolic prophylaxis

Sick patients with IE are frequently bedbound, increasing the risk of deep venous thrombosis and pulmonary embolism. Appropriate prevention strategies include compression stockings and prophylactic heparin. Careful assessment of the balance of risks and benefits of anticoagulation may be required in patients with neurological complications or high bleeding risk.

Education and emotional support

Many patients face a long period of treatment with uncertain outcome. Depression is common. Care must be taken to provide sufficient information and education regarding the disease and its treatment. Early prosthetic valve IE can be emotionally devastating, particularly if re-do surgery is likely. Early involvement of family members and other carers is essential.

Home therapy and follow up

Many patients with uncomplicated IE are able to receive the latter part of their treatment at home, if appropriate support and health care facilities exist. Early discussion and planning should involve the patient's primary care team and access to appropriate follow up and specialist advice.

Surgical centre referral

Many patients with uncomplicated native valve IE can be safely managed in a hospital without direct access to cardiac surgery. However, early communication and discussion with a surgical centre is advised in all but the most straightforward cases. This may involve transfer of the patient for assessment and a period of monitoring.

Patients requiring early transfer to a surgical centre include:
• Confirmed IE with evidence of progression or new complication, e.g. new heart block or embolic event
• Prosthetic valve IE
• Complications likely to require surgery
• Failure of early medical therapy
• Uncertain diagnosis—further imaging may be required.

There is nothing to be lost by discussion and early referral. Transfer of a stable patient who does not ultimately need surgery is preferable to delay until a critical state emerges, when the risks of intervention become prohibitive.

Additional pathology

Streptococcus bovis infection is associated with colonic malignancy in around 20% of patients. All such patients should undergo colonoscopy screening during or after medical therapy with repeat assessment at six months if initial investigation is negative.

Intravenous drug users should be screened for hepatitis and HIV after appropriate discussion and informed consent.

Empirical medical therapy

Prompt treatment of IE is critical (although not at the expense of correctly performed blood cultures). Once appropriate cultures have been acquired, it may be appropriate to commence empirical antibiotic therapy until the organism has been identified. In many stable patients, however, delaying treatment for 24–48 hours is unlikely to be harmful and allows guided therapy from the outset.

The choice of empirical therapy depends on three factors:
- Use of prior antibiotic therapy.
- Native or prosthetic valve IE (early vs. late).
- Local epidemiology and antibiotic resistance.

Empirical therapy for native valve infective endocarditis

Regimes for native valve IE must cover staphylococci, streptococci, HACEK organisms, and *Bartonella* species. An appropriate regime is (assumed weight 75kg):
- Amoxicillin 3g IV every 6 hours   12g/day
  with
- Gentamicin 80mg IV/IM every 8 hours   3mg/kg/day

An alternative regime for penicillin-allergic patients is:
- Vancomycin 1g IV every 12 hours   30mg/kg/day
  with
- Gentamicin 80mg IV/IM every 8 hours   3mg/kg/day
  with
- Ciprofloxacin 400mg IV every 12 hours   800mg/day

Doxycycline may also be added if *Bartonella* infection is suspected (classically seen in homeless patients).

Empirical therapy for prosthetic valve infective endocarditis

Treatment for early prosthetic valve IE (<12 months since surgery) must cover Methicillin resistant *Staphylococcus aureus* (MRSA) and non-HACEK Gram-negative pathogens. An appropriate regime is (assumed weight 75kg):
- Vancomycin 1g IV every 12 hours   30mg/kg/day
  with
- Gentamicin 80mg IV/IM every 8 hours   3mg/kg/day
  with
- Rifampicin 600mg PO every 12 hours   1200mg/day

Empirical therapy for late prosthetic valve infective endocarditis

The spectrum of organisms in late prosthetic valve endocarditis mirrors that of native valve infection. Empirical management follows the same regime as for native valve IE until further microbiological data are available.

Antimicrobial therapy

The aims of treatment are to control infection, prevent progression, and sterilize the valve and adherent vegetations. Prolonged intravenous therapy is usually required (2–6 weeks, and sometimes longer), the precise regime depending on many factors, including the organism and its sensitivity. Microbiological advice should always be sought.

Treatment is deemed to start on the first day of effective antimicrobial therapy (the initial regime may be extensively modified in the light of microbiological findings). This clock does not restart at the time of surgery unless there is evidence of uncontrolled infection or remaining viable organisms at the time of microscopy and culture of the excised valve.

The following regimes are recommended in streptococcal and staphylococcal IE (assumed patient weight 75kg). Exact treatment may vary according to local guidelines, available antibiotics and the results of microbiological testing.

Streptococcus infective endocarditis treatment regimes:

Streptococcal IE:

Fully penicillin-sensitive strains

4–6 weeks of:

- Benzylpenicillin 1.2g IV every 4 hours   12–18million U/day
  or
- Amoxicillin 2g IV every 4 hours   100–200mg/kg/day
  or
- Ceftriaxone 2g IV/IM every 24 hours
  or
- Vancomycin 1g IV every 12 hours   30mg/kg/day.

Shorter regimes using the synergistic effects of an aminoglycoside are possible in uncomplicated native valve IE:

2 weeks of Benzylpenicillin, amoxicillin or Ceftriaxone (as above) plus two weeks of either:

- Gentamicin 225mg IV/IM every 24 hours   3mg/kg/day
  or
- Netilmicin 375mg IV every 24 hours   4 – 5mg/kg/day.

Relatively penicillin resistant strains
An additional aminoglycoside is required.

4–6 weeks of:
- Benzylpenicillin 2.4g IV every 4 hours   24 million U/day
  or
- Amoxicillin 2.5g IV every 4 hours   200mg/kg/day
  with

2 weeks of:
- Gentamicin 225mg IV/IM every 24 hours   3mg/kg/day

An alternative regime in penicillin-allergic patients is:
- Vancomycin 1g IV every 12 hours   30mg/kg/day
  with
- Gentamicin 225mg IV/IM every 24 hours   3mg/kg/day

Monitoring and drug levels

Renal function should be monitored at least twice weekly when Gentamicin, Netilmicin or Vancomycin are used. Drug levels should also be monitored to avoid toxicity and ensure that therapeutic levels are achieved. Note that ototoxicity is common, difficult to detect in the hospital environment and often overlooked.

Gentamicin: trough level <1mg/L, 1 hour post-dose peak 10-12mg/L.

Vancomycin: trough level 10–15mg/L, 1 hour post-dose peak 30-45mg/L.

Staphylococcal IE

Methicillin-susceptible staphylococci: native valve

If the organism is confirmed to be a sensitive staphylococcus (i.e. MSSA *not* MRSA) then the following regime can be used:

4–6 weeks of either:
- Flucloxacillin 2g IV every 4 hours   12g/day
             or
- Oxacillin 2g IV every 4 hours   12g/day
             with

3–5 days of:
- Gentamicin 80mg IV/IM every 8 hours   3mg/kg/day.

Treat as Methicillin-resistant staphylococcal IE if the patient is allergic to β-lactam penicillin.

Methicillin-resistant staphylococci: native valve

If the organism is confirmed to be a resistant staphylococcus (i.e. MRSA) (or if the patient is allergic to penicillin) then the following regime is appropriate:

At least 6 weeks of:
- Vancomycin 1g IV every 12 hours   30mg/kg/day
             with

3–5 days of:
- Gentamicin 80mg IV/IM every 8 hours   3mg/kg/day.

Staphylococcal IE: prosthetic valve

Prosthetic valve IE requires additional treatment with Rifampicin which has particular effects on infected prosthetic material. Gentamicin therapy is also extended to two weeks.

The regime is the same as for native valvular heart disease but with the addition of:

At least 6 weeks of:
- Rifampicin 600mg IV/PO every 12 hours   1200mg/day

Monitoring and drug levels

The recommended levels of Gentamicin and Vancomycin are the same as in streptococcal infection. Rifampicin and Flucloxacillin are associated with deranged liver function which may influence the metabolism of other drugs, e.g. warfarin. Frequent monitoring is required.

Enterococcal IE

Enterococci are often resistant to antimicrobial therapy and prolonged therapy may be required.

Treatment regimes for sensitive strains include:

4–6 weeks of both:
- Amoxicillin 2.5g IV every 4 hours   200mg/kg/day
    and
- Gentamicin 80mg IV/IM every 8 hours   3mg/kg/day
    or

4–6 weeks of both:
- Vancomycin 1g IV every 12 hours   30mg/kg/day
    and
- Gentamicin 80mg IV/IM every 8 hours   3mg/kg/day.

Monitoring and drug levels

Special attention is warranted in view of the longer duration of gentamicin therapy.

HACEK IE

These organisms (see 📖 p.360) are difficult to treat and early expert microbiological advice should be sought early. A suggested regime is:

4 weeks of:
- Ceftriaxone 2g IV/IM every 24 hours.

If susceptibility to β-lactam penicillin is demonstrated then an alternative regime is:

4 weeks of both:
- Ampicillin 2g IV every 4 hours   12g/day
    and
- Gentamicin 80mg IV/IM every 8 hours   3mg/kg/day.

Non-HACEK Gram-negative IE

This rare situation requires a combination of early surgery and expert microbiological advice. Combinations of penicillin, gentamicin, and cotrimoxazole (or ciprofloxacin) may be required.

Prosthetic valve infective endocarditis

Around 25% of all cases of IE involve a prosthetic valve—mechanical valves and bioprostheses are equally affected.

Diagnosis is often difficult as a result of subtle clinical signs and issues with imaging the prosthesis and its surrounding tissues. Eradication of infection is also more challenging. Prognosis is therefore poor and in-hospital mortality may be as high as 40%.

Infection may be defined as early (within one year of surgery) or late (>1 year since surgery). Early prosthetic valve endocarditis usually arises as a result of contamination during surgery or haematogenous spread affecting the sewing ring and sutures. Staphylococcal infection is frequent, leading to early abscess formation and valve dehiscence (Fig. 16.9). The microbiology and pathophysiology of late prosthetic valve endocarditis resemble native valve disease.

Conventional diagnostic criteria apply, although blood cultures are more frequently negative and the sensitivity of transoesophageal echocardiography is reduced. Clinical assessment in the early post-operative period may also be hampered by the presence of alternative explanations for fever. Antimicrobial regimes used in native valve IE apply, though prolonged regimes and additional Rifampicin may be required.

Surgery for prosthetic valve infective endocarditis

High risk redo surgery is frequently required, particularly for early infection, and should be actively considered in the following situations:
- Heart failure refractory to medical therapy
- Uncontrolled infection—abscess formation or enlarging vegetation
- Staphylococcal or fungal infection
- Resistant organism or persistent infection (fever and positive cultures) after seven days treatment
- Recurrent embolic events despite medical therapy
- Severe prosthetic dehiscence (even if well tolerated).

Patients with refractory pulmonary oedema or cardiogenic shock are extremely challenging and may require immediate life-saving surgery.

The surgical principles in prosthetic valve endocarditis are as follows:
- Debridement of all infected material
- Removal of calcified areas which may be infected
- Root replacement if involved in aortic prosthetic valve endocarditis (homograft or xenograft may be used)
- Restoration of atrioventricular continuity (patch repair if required)
- Valve replacement—choice of prosthesis depends on surgical factors (see 📖 p.266) but use of prosthetic material should be minimized.

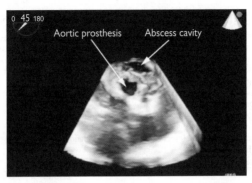

Fig. 16.9 3D transoesophageal echocardiogram demonstrating an extensive abscess cavity posterior to the sewing ring of a bioprosthetic aortic valve.

Culture negative infective endocarditis

The rate of culture negative IE varies considerably, but can be as high as 30% of all cases. The diagnosis is defined by a clinical diagnosis of IE without an identifiable organism in at least three separate blood cultures after seven days. Negative blood cultures in a patient with a high clinical likelihood of IE can occur for several reasons:

• Previous antimicrobial administration—particularly if sensitive organism (e.g. streptococcus)
• Inappropriate or inadequate culture techniques
• Non-bacterial pathogen (e.g. fungus)
• Fastidious bacterial infection requiring prolonged culture or specialised techniques.

Potential unusual organisms in culture negative IE include:

Organism	Potential treatment
Coxiella burnetii	Doxycycline and Ofloxacin (at least 18 months)
Bartonella spp.	Ceftriaxone (6 weeks) and Gentamicin (3 weeks)
Brucella spp.	Doxycycline, cotrimoxazole and Rifampicin (at least 3 months)
Tropheryma whipplei	Doxycycline and hydroxychloroquine (long term)
Mycoplasma hominis	Quinolone, e.g. moxifloxacin (long term)
Legionella pneumophilia	Erythromycin and ciprofloxacin (6 weeks total)

Culture negative IE is more likely in patients with prosthetic valves, ind-welling prosthetic material, and impaired immunity. If suspected, microbiological advice should be sought and blood sent for appropriate serological testing. Similarly, if surgery is undertaken for culture negative IE then excised material should be sent for:

• Tissue culture—fastidious bacteria may be grown with prolonged culture and specialized techniques
• Histopathology—viable and non-viable organisms may be identified
• Immunohistology—detection of organism-specific antigens
• Polymerase chain reaction—bacterial DNA may be identified.

Right-sided infective endocarditis

Primary involvement of the tricuspid (or rarely pulmonary) valves is observed in about 10% of cases. Some relate to the presence of intravenous catheters or pacemaker leads, but the majority arise in intravenous drug users.

These patients are often malnourished and immunosuppressed (some with human immunodeficiency virus [HIV] infection). Injection of impure solutions containing particulate material may cause primary injury to the valve endothelium and needle contamination (often with skin commensals) leads to bacteraemia. Staphylococci are the most frequently encountered organisms and infections with fungi and Gram-negative bacteria are also seen.

The general features of IE (notably fever and bacteraemia) remain but embolic complications affect the pulmonary bed. Patients may therefore present with a primary respiratory illness characterized by multiple pulmonary abscesses and infarction with subsequent empyema.

Heart failure is a rare complication unless valve destruction leads to severe tricuspid or PR. Right heart failure may also develop as a consequence of severe pulmonary infection/infarction with secondary pulmonary hypertension. Prognosis is good unless there are very large vegetations (Fig. 16.10), fungal infection, or background HIV-associated immune compromise.

Empirical therapy should address staphylococci (including MRSA), pseudomonal and fungal infections (including *Candida*).

Intravenous access can be challenging (and may be abused) in this cohort. Oral treatment regimes should only be contemplated in compliant patients with staphylococcal infection fully sensitive to quinolones and rifampicin.

Surgery is rarely required, but should be considered in the following settings:

• Persistent infection despite appropriate medical therapy against a resistant organism (e.g. *Pseudomonas aeruginosa*, fungi)
• Persistent large vegetation (>20mm) and recurrent pulmonary emboli
• Refractory right heart failure due to severe tricuspid or PR.

The risk of recurrent IE is high unless abstinence from further intravenous drug use can be guaranteed. If surgery is required, conservative techniques (vegetation excision and valve repair) are preferred and homografts may play a role.

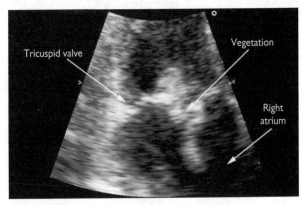

Fig. 16.10 Transthoracic echocardiogram of the tricuspid valve demonstrating a large pedunculated vegetation prolapsing into both the RV and right atrium.

Device-related infective endocarditis

The number of implanted pacemakers and defibrillators is steadily increasing and the rate of infection of these devices is at least 1–2 per 1000 device years. This frequency is likely to climb as indications widen and more box change and revision procedures are required. The extent of device-related infection can range from a superficial wound or subcutaneous pocket infection to frank sepsis involving the device, electrodes (leads) and endocardium. Approximately 50% of cases of device related IE have valvular (usually tricuspid) involvement.

Infection relates to direct contamination at the time of implantation with subsequent spread along the electrodes, or haematogenous spread from a remote site with seeding on the electrode. Prophylactic antibiotics at the time of implantation reduce infection rates and particular care is required in patients requiring temporary transvenous pacing or device implantation in the presence of active infection.

Infection is a particular risk during revision procedures, especially device upgrades when additional electrodes may be introduced. Additional risk factors include diabetes, anticoagulation (with increasing bleeding), age, operator inexperience, surgical technique, and duration of procedure. Staphylococci (especially *Staphylococcus aureus*) are the most commonly involved organisms.

Diagnosis

A very high index of suspicion is required since patients often present with vague symptoms and few specific clinical signs. Fever is common (but less marked in the elderly or immunosuppressed) and local infection may be suggested by tenderness or inflammation of the device pocket.

Early echocardiography may identify vegetations on the electrodes (Fig. 16.11), tricuspid valve, or endocardium, but not in the superior vena cava, subclavian, or axillary vein. Transoesophageal imaging is superior and recommended in all patients with suspected device related IE.

However, even a negative study does not fully exclude the diagnosis. As in right sided IE, embolism of infected material to the pulmonary circulation is a common complication. Device-related IE must be excluded in any patient with an implanted pacemaker or defibrillator presenting with a primary respiratory illness.

Management

Percutaneous removal of the device and electrodes with subsequent prolonged antibiotic therapy is the only effective treatment option. Procedures are often difficult with risk of cardiac perforation and a surgical approach is occasionally necessary. The timing of extraction and re-implantation (if indicated) is case-dependent and specialist input is recommended.

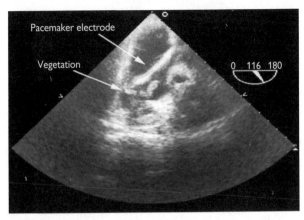

Fig. 16.11 Transoesophageal echocardiogram demonstrating a large vegetation adherent to a pacing electrode in the right atrium.

Antimicrobial therapy

Antimicrobial therapy is guided by culture of blood, tissue swabs and any explanted material. Empirical therapy should target staphylococci (including MRSA). A suggested regime is:

4–6 weeks of:
- Vancomycin 1g IV every 12 hours   30mg/kg/day
  with
- Gentamicin 80mg IV/IM every 8 hours   3mg/kg/day
  and
- Rifampicin 600mg PO every 12 hours   1200mg/day

Additional points

- Treatment with prolonged medical therapy alone is occasionally successful. This strategy is rarely appropriate in view of the high likelihood of eventual relapse
- Device extraction should be considered in patients with a pacemaker or defibrillator and unexplained recurrent bacteraemia
- All device procedures (including 'simple' box-changes) should be performed by experienced operators using meticulous surgical technique and appropriate antibiotic prophylaxis
- Erosion of a device through the skin is often a manifestation of infection. Explantation is usually recommended.

Surgical therapy

Surgery for IE is performed to achieve three goals:
• Complete removal of infected tissue
• Restoration of normal cardiac anatomy and valve function
• Reversal of haemodynamic abnormalities.

Nearly half of all patients with IE require surgery at some point. Timing is often difficult and indications range between from immediate intervention to prevent death from acute heart failure, early surgery for complications and later correction of residual valve dysfunction.

At all times, the decision to operate requires careful collaboration between the cardiologist, cardiac surgeon, anaesthetic team, and microbiologist to determine the relative risks and benefits of surgical intervention and ongoing medical therapy.

Indications for early surgery in IE include:
• Heart failure refractory to medical therapy
• Uncontrolled infection despite appropriate medical therapy
• High risk of embolism
• Early prosthetic valve endocarditis
• Infection with resistant or aggressive organisms
  • Fungi – high embolic potential
  • Multiresistant Gram-positive cocci
  • *Coxiella burnetii*
  • *Brucella*
  • *Pseudomonas aeruginosa*.

Heart failure due to infective endocarditis

Heart failure is the most common cause of death in IE and the most frequent indication for surgery. Severe AR or MR as a result of valve destruction is the most frequent cause although heart failure may also rarely arise as a result of fistulae, valve obstruction by large vegetations, or right-sided valvular heart disease.

Initial medical management is targeted at the maintenance of adequate end-organ perfusion and oxygenation. These patients are often complex and additional co-morbidities, e.g. renal failure, pre-existing LV dysfunction, and the haemodynamic effects of septicaemia can complicate the clinical picture. Management by a specialist team is recommended.

Uncontrolled infection in infective endocarditis

Uncontrolled infection implies appropriate antimicrobial therapy for >7 days with evidence of persisting fever or progressive infection.

Persistent fever

A number of possibilities must be excluded before treatment failure is declared:

- Inadequate or inappropriate antimicrobial therapy
  - Are the correct weight adjusted doses being used?
  - Have therapeutic levels been achieved?
  - Is the organism sensitive to the chosen regime?
  - Are additional drugs (e.g. Rifampicin) affecting metabolism?
- Additional source of infection
  - Intravenous line related infection?
  - Pneumonia complicating embolic event or prolonged immobility?
  - Urinary infection complicating catheter insertion?
  - 'Missed' portal of entry of original infection—skin or teeth?
- Embolic complications
  - Solid organ abscess formation—spleen/kidneys/brain?
  - Spinal infection—discitis?
  - Osteomyelitis?
- Drug related
  - Hypersensitivity reaction?
  - Pyrogenic contaminants in drugs or fluids?
  - Chemical phlebitis?
- Other rare causes:
  - Thyroid disturbance
  - Pulmonary embolism
  - Neuroleptic malignant syndrome (anaesthetic agents)
  - Connective tissue disease.

Progressive infection

Perivalvar extension of infection leading to abscess formation (with potential progression to pseudoaneurysm or fistula formation) is a common feature of both native aortic valve and prosthetic valve IE. These complications carry a high risk of mortality, even if surgery is undertaken (Fig. 16.12).

Serial transoesophageal imaging to exclude abscess should be undertaken in any patient not responding adequately to medical therapy. A further helpful sign is progressive lengthening of the PR interval as a result of local disruption of the conduction system. Development of pericardial pain or a new pericardial effusion may reflect abscess progression beyond the aortic root and is equally concerning.

Increasing vegetation size despite adequate antimicrobial treatment also suggests uncontrolled infection and confers a higher risk of subsequent embolic complications.

High risk for embolic events

Embolic events occur in up to 50% of patients with IE. The brain is most frequently affected and approximately one third of events are clinically silent. The risk of embolism falls dramatically following initiation of medical therapy, particularly after the first 7–10 days of treatment.

Factors predicting the risk of embolism include:
- Large (>10mm) or very large (>15mm) vegetations
- Markedly mobile vegetations
- Mitral valve involvement
- Increasing vegetation size despite medical therapy
- Staphylococcal IE.

Repeat transoesophageal echocardiography and consideration of surgery is appropriate in a patient with recurrent embolism after 5–7 days of appropriate medical treatment. The presence of a very large (>15mm) vegetation is also considered an indication for surgery in some centres (particularly if valve conserving surgery is likely).

In reality, surgery is rarely justified based upon vegetation size alone, but a combination of factors (large vegetation, aggressive organism, e.g. *Staphylococcus aureus*, significant valvular regurgitation) which collectively indicate surgery frequently coexists in such patients. Early multidisciplinary discussion and close surveillance with serial imaging are always appropriate.

Preventing embolic events

Anticoagulation increases the likelihood of bleeding complications in IE and has no systematic role in the prevention of embolism. If indicated for other reasons, e.g. mechanical valve or high risk atrial fibrillation, then anticoagulants should be used with extreme care, particularly with regard to interactions with antimicrobial agents.

Limited evidence suggests some benefit of anti-platelet therapy in this setting, presumably secondary to modified platelet aggregation during vegetation formation. However, routine use of these agents is not yet recommended.

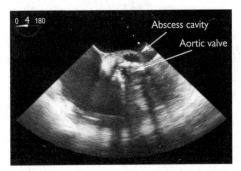

Fig. 16.12 Transoesophageal echocardiogram demonstrating gross abnormalities of the aortic root and a large posterior abscess cavity complicating *Staphylococcus Aureus* prosthetic valve endocarditis.

Antimicrobial therapy post surgery

The recommended course of treatment starts on the first day of appropriate adequate antimicrobial therapy and NOT the day of cardiac surgery. This clock is not reset unless culture of excised material demonstrates viable bacteria. In patients undergoing surgery towards the end of their course of antibiotic therapy, it is prudent to continue treatment until the outcome of microbiological investigations is available.

Outcomes of surgery

Overall mortality is approximately 5–15% following surgery for IE, but is higher (10–30%) for patients with prosthetic valve endocarditis (recurrent infection remains an issue and affects up to 15% of patients). Individual outcomes vary according to preoperative clinical status, co-morbidity, extent of infection, duration of surgery, and experience of the operator and surgical team.

Management of complications

Extra-cardiac complications of IE are frequent and have a major influence on outcome. Early involvement of appropriate specialists and regular multidisciplinary discussions are key to successful management.

It is also important to recognise that patients may initially present to non-cardiac disciplines with symptoms and signs of an underlying complication of IE. Vigilance and a low index of suspicion (especially in high risk groups) are vital.

Neurological complications

Embolism of infected debris to the cerebral circulation can lead to a range of neurological sequelae:
- Stroke or transient ischaemic attack
- Meningoencephalitis
- Meningitis
- Mycotic aneurysm
- Intra-cranial haemorrhage
  - ruptured mycotic aneurysm
  - bleeding into cerebral infarction
- Cerebral abscess
- Seizure—secondary to any of the above
- Spinal injury complicating embolism to the spinal vessels
- Spinal injury complicating disc infection
- Epidural abscess.

Cardiac surgery following neurological injury

A frequent clinical dilemma is the timing of cardiac surgery for IE in a patient with a recent neurological complication. The prime concern is the risk of bleeding into recently injured neurological tissue. Such surgery should only be undertaken after careful multidisciplinary discussion and weighting of the relative risks and benefits. General considerations include:
- Cardiac surgery is safe in patients with a recent embolic stroke or transient ischaemic attack and no evidence of cerebral haemorrhage, abscess, or meningitis
- Cardiac surgery should be delayed by at least four weeks following cerebral haemorrhage if possible. Successful early surgical intervention has been reported, particularly if the risk of further bleeding can be reduced (e.g. by coil exclusion of a solitary mycotic aneurysm)
- Cardiac surgery should not be contemplated if the outcome of neurological injury is likely to be severe
- Cardiac surgery should not be contemplated in patients with severe co-morbidities or persistent coma.

Renal complications

Acute renal failure is encountered in one third of patients and associated with adverse outcome. Aetiology is often multifactorial but potential causes include:

- Glomerulonephritis—immune complex mediated (common with *Staphylococcus aureus* and the viridans *Streptococci*)
- Interstitial nephritis—due to penicillin, quinolone, or cephalosporin
- Acute tubular necrosis—may be caused by gentamicin
- Renal embolism—may lead to secondary abscess formation
- Hypoperfusion—as a consequence of haemodynamic instability
- Nephrotoxicity—contrast media for CT or coronary angiography.

Management relies on supportive measures which may include short term renal replacement therapy. Modified antibiotic regimes may be required. Maintenance of optimal fluid balance in a patient with valvular regurgitation, heart failure, and evolving renal failure is challenging and often requires invasive monitoring in a high-dependency or intensive care environment.

Other complications

Abscesses in solid organs (e.g. the spleen) are often silent and can lead to persistent fever and apparent treatment failure. Splenectomy is occasionally required and should be undertaken before cardiac surgery to avoid postoperative valve re-infection.

Joint collections and septic arthritis may be the initial presenting feature of IE.

Adverse effects of high dose antimicrobial therapy and prolonged hospital stay include:

- Ototoxicity
- Nephrotoxicity
- Hepatic dysfunction
- Bone marrow suppression
- Venous thromboembolism
- Pressure sores
- Nosocomial infections
- Psychosocial problems.

Infective endocarditis prophylaxis

Previous widespread (and sometimes indiscriminate) use of antibiotic prophylaxis prior to medical or dental procedures to reduce risk of IE has recently been questioned. Major revisions to national and international guidelines are based on a number of key principles:

- There is scant evidence to support the use of antibiotic prophylaxis to prevent IE and no randomized controlled studies
- Transient bacteraemia is common during daily activities, e.g. tooth brushing and occurs spontaneously in patients with poor oral hygiene
- There is little consistent evidence for significant bacteraemia arising as a result of medical or dental procedures
- The number requiring antibiotic prophylaxis to prevent one case of IE is in the many thousands
- Only a minority of patients with IE have an obvious index event causing potentially preventable bacteraemia
- Antibiotic administration carries a small risk of anaphylaxis and a higher risk of promoting resistant organisms
- IE frequently arises in patients with no known history of cardiac disease in whom routine prophylaxis would be inapplicable
- The epidemiology of IE is changing and episodes related to dental flora are increasingly infrequent.

Counter arguments are based on the knowledge and experience that IE is a devastating, potentially fatal disease, even with modern treatment. However, it is clear that widespread use of antibiotic prophylaxis will only influence outcome in a very small number of patients. In the UK, the National Institute for Health and Clinical Excellence have recommended that the practice of antibiotic prophylaxis is abandoned altogether. Guidelines in Europe and the USA continue to recommend prophylaxis in high risk groups.

General measures

Updated guidelines have emphasised general measures to prevent IE:
- Meticulous oral hygiene and regular dental checks.
- Avoidance of tattoos and piercing procedures.
- Education and awareness of the symptoms of IE.
- Prompt assessment and treatment of infection in at risk patients.
- Avoidance of unnecessary invasive procedures (e.g. cannula insertion or urinary catheterisation) in at risk patients.
- Strict sterile technique during invasive procedures—in particular central venous catheter insertion.

Specific prophylactic measures

Current European guidelines recommend antibiotic prophylaxis in the following circumstances:
- Patient at high risk of IE *and*
- Procedure with high risk of causing IE.

High risk patients

A cumulative risk of both the likelihood of acquiring IE and higher attendant mortality and morbidity:
- Prosthetic valves of any type
- Prosthetic material for cardiac repair
- Patients with previous IE (even if treated successfully)
- Complex cyanotic congenital heart disease (particularly if remaining surgical shunts, conduits or other prosthetic material).

Patients not requiring prophylaxis

The following groups do not require prophylaxis for any procedure:
- Bicuspid aortic valve disease
- AS or AR
- MS or MR
- Mitral valve prolapse
- Hypertrophic cardiomyopathy.

High risk procedures

The following procedures carry the highest risk of causing IE:
- Dental procedures requiring gingival manipulation or perforation of oral mucosa
- Implantation of cardiac or vascular prosthesis or other foreign material.

Patients at high risk of IE undergoing invasive procedures for established infection (respiratory, gastrointestinal or genitourinary tract, skin or musculoskeletal system) should receive an antibiotic regime which covers potential IE-causative organisms.

Recommended prophylactic regime

If high risk criteria are met then the patient should receive the following regime 30–60 minutes before the procedure:
- Amoxicillin 2g PO/IV (or same dose Ampicillin)
  or (if penicillin allergic):
- Clindamycin 600mg PO/IV.

Algorithm for echocardiography in suspected infective endocarditis

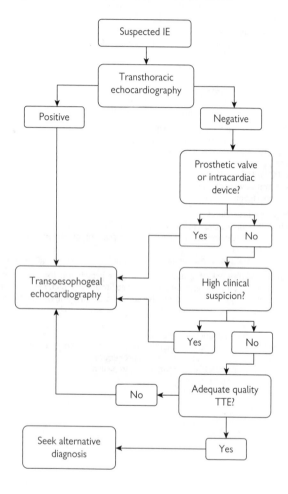

Further reading

Listed below are selected references on valvular heart disease relevant to each chapter of this book.

Chapter 1 Introduction to valvular heart disease

Iung B., Baron G., Butchart E.G., Delahaye F., Gohlke-Barwolf C., Levang O.W., Tornos P., Vanoverschelde J.-L., Vermeer F., Boersma E., Ravaud P., Vahanian A. (2003) A prospective survey of patients with valvular heart disease in Europe: The Euro Heart Survey on Valvular Heart Disease. *Eur. Heart J.* 24(13):1231–1243.

Ho S.Y. (2002) Anatomy of the mitral valve. *Heart* 88: 5–10.

Ho S.Y. (2009) Structure and anatomy of the aortic root. *Eur. J. Echocardiogr.* 10(1):i3–10.

Chapter 2 Assessment of valvular heart disease

Zoghbi W. (2003) Recommendations for evaluation of the severity of native valvular regurgitation with two-dimensional and Doppler echocardiography. *J. Am. Soc. Echocardiogr.* 16:777–802.

Eugenio P., Philippe P., Patrizio L., Jean Luc M., Robert O.B. (2009) The Emerging Role of Exercise Testing and Stress Echocardiography in Valvular Heart Disease. *J. Am. Coll. Cardiol.* 54(24):2251–2260.

Baumgartner H., Hung J., Bermejo J., Chambers J.B., Evangelista A., Griffin B.P., Iung B., Otto C.M., Pellikka P.A., Quinones M. (2009) Echocardiographic assessment of valve stenosis: EAE/ASE recommendations for clinical practice. *Eur. J. Echocardiogr.* 10(1):1–25.

Chapter 3 General management

Iung B., Gohlke-Barwolf C., Tornos P., Tribouilloy C., Hall R., Butchart E., Vahanian A. Recommendations on the management of the asymptomatic patient with valvular heart disease. (2002) *Eur. Heart J.* 23(16):1253–1266.

Rahimtoola S.H. (2003) Choice of prosthetic heart valve for adult patients. *J. Am. Coll. Cardiol.* 41(6):893–904.

Chapter 4 Aortic stenosis

Vahanian A., Otto C.M. Risk stratification of patients with aortic stenosis. *Eur. Heart J.* 31(4) 416–423.

Rosenhek R., Zilberszac R., Schemper M., Czerny M., Mundigler G., Graf S., Bergler-Klein J., Grimm M., Gabriel H., Maurer G. Natural History of Very Severe Aortic Stenosis. *Circulation* 121(1) 151–156.

Otto C. (2006) Valvular aortic stenosis: Disease severity and timing of intervention. *J. Am Coll. Cardiol.* 47: 2141–2151.

Otto C.M. (2000) Aortic Stenosis: Listen to the Patient, Look at the Valve. *N. Engl. J. Med.* 343(9):652–654.

Dumesnil J.G., Pibarot P., Carabello B. Paradoxical low flow and/or low gradient severe aortic stenosis despite preserved left ventricular ejection fraction: implications for diagnosis and treatment. *Eur. Heart J.* 31(3):281–289.

Chapter 5 Aortic regurgitation

Choudhry N. (1999) Does this patient have aortic regurgitation? *J. Am. Med. Assoc.* 28:2231–2238.

Maurer G. (2006) Aortic regurgitation. *Heart* 92:994–1000.

Bekeredjian R., Grayburn P.A. (2005) Valvular Heart Disease: Aortic Regurgitation. *Circulation* 112(1):125–134.

Chapter 6 Mitral stenosis

Chandrashekhar Y., Westaby S., Narula J. (2009) Mitral stenosis. *Lancet* 374(9697):1271–83.

Carabello B. (2005) Modern management of mitral stenosis. *Circulation* 11:432–437.

Turgeman Y. (2003) Subvalvular apparatus in rheumatic mitral stenosis. *Chest* 12:1929–1936.

Chapter 7 Mitral regurgitation

Di Salvo T.G., Acker M.A., Dec G.W., Byrne J.G. Mitral Valve Surgery in Advanced Heart Failure. *J. Am. Coll. Cardiol.* 55(4):271–282.

Enriquez-Sarano M. (2003) Mitral regurgitation: what causes the leakage is fundamental to the outcome of valve repair. *Circulation* 10:253–256.

Griffin B. (2006) Timing of surgical intervention in chronic mitral regurgitation: is vigilance enough? *Circulation* 11:2169–2172.

Irvine T. (2002) Assessment of mitral regurgitation. *Heart supplement* 88:11–19.

Iung B. (2003) Management of ischaemic mitral regurgitation. *Heart* 89 (4): 459–464.

Otto C. (2003) Timing of surgery in mitral regurgitation. *Heart* 89:100–105.

Rosenhek R. (2006) Outcome of watchful waiting in asymptomatic severe mitral regurgitation. *Circulation* 11:2328–2344.

Unger P., Dedobbeleer C., Van Camp G., Plein D., Cosyns B., Lancellotti P. (2009) Mitral regurgitation in patients with aortic stenosis undergoing valve replacement. *Heart*: 165548.

Chapter 8 Tricuspid stenosis

Waller B.F., Howard J., Fess S. Pathology of tricuspid valve stenosis and pure tricuspid regurgitation Part I. (1995) *Clin. Cardiol.* 18(2):97–102.

Chapter 9 Tricuspid regurgitation

Antunes M.J. (2007) Management of tricuspid valve regurgitation. *Heart* 93:271–276.

Chapter 10 Pulmonary stenosis

Lurz P., Coats L., Khambadkone S., Nordmeyer J., Boudjemline Y., Schievano S., Muthurangu V., Lee T.Y., Parenzan G., Derrick G., Cullen S., Walker F., Tsang V., Deanfield J., Taylor A.M., Bonhoeffer P. (2008) Percutaneous Pulmonary Valve Implantation: Impact of Evolving Technology and Learning Curve on Clinical Outcome. *Circulation* 117(15):1964–1972.

Chapter 11 Pulmonary regurgitation

Bouzas B., Kilner P.J., Gatzoulis M.A.(2005) Pulmonary regurgitation: not a benign lesion. *Eur. Heart J.* 26(5):433–439.

Chapter 12 Surgery and prosthetic valves

Verma S., Mesana T.G. (2009) Mitral-Valve Repair for Mitral-Valve Prolapse. *N. Engl. J. Med.* 361(23):2261–2269.

Di Salvo T.G., Acker M.A., Dec G.W., Byrne J.G. Mitral Valve Surgery in Advanced Heart Failure. *J. Am. Coll. Cardiol.* 55(4):271–282.

William A.Z., John B.C., Jean G.D., Elyse F., John S.G., Paul A.G., Bijoy K.K., Robert A.L., Gerald Ross M., Fletcher A.M., Satoshi N., Miguel A.Qo, Harry R., Rodriguez L.L., Madhav S., Alan D.W., Neil J.W., Miguel Z. (2009) Recommendations for Evaluation of Prosthetic Valves With Echocardiography and Doppler Ultrasound: A Report From the American Society of Echocardiography's Guidelines and Standards Committee and the Task Force on Prosthetic Valves. *J. Am. Soc. Echocardiogr.* 22(9):975–1014.

Chapter 13 Percutaneous valve therapy

Feldman T. (2005) Percutaneous mitral valve repair with the edge-to-edge technique - EVEREST trial. *J. Am. Coll. Cardiol.* 46:2134–2140.

Grube E., Schuler G., Buellesfeld L., Gerckens U., Linke A., Wenaweser P., Sauren B., Mohr F.-W., Walther T., Zickmann B., Iversen S., Felderhoff T., Cartier R., Bonan R. (2007) Percutaneous Aortic Valve Replacement for Severe Aortic Stenosis in High-Risk Patients Using the Second- and Current Third-Generation Self-Expanding CoreValve Prosthesis: Device Success and 30-Day Clinical Outcome. *J. Am. Coll. Cardiol.* 50(1):69–76.

Munt B. (2006) Percutaneous valve repair and replacement techniques. *Heart* 92: 1369–1372.

Chapter 14 Management during non-cardiac surgery

Authors/Task Force Members, Poldermans D., Bax J.J., Boersma E., De Hert S., Eeckhout E., Fowkes G., Gorenek B., Hennerici M.G., Iung B., Kelm M., Kjeldsen K.P., Kristensen S.D., Lopez-Sendon J., Pelosi P., Philippe F., Pierard L., Ponikowski P., Schmid J.-P., Sellevold O.F.M., Sicari R., Van den Berghe G., Vermassen F., Additional Contributors, Hoeks S.E., Vanhorebeek I. (2009) ESC. Guidelines for pre-operative cardiac risk assessment and perioperative cardiac management in non-cardiac surgery: The Task Force for Preoperative Cardiac Risk Assessment and Perioperative Cardiac Management in Non-cardiac Surgery of the European Society of Cardiology (ESC) and endorsed by the European Society of Anaesthesiology (ESA). *Eur Heart J.* 30(22):2769–2812.

Chapter 15 Valvular heart disease in pregnancy

Stout K.K., Otto C.M. (2007) Pregnancy in women with valvular heart disease. *Heart* 93(5): 552–558.

Elkayam U. (2005) Valvular heart disease in pregnancy - prosthetic valves. *J. Am. Coll. Cardiol.* 46:403–410.

Elkayam U, Bitar F. (2005) Valvular Heart Disease and Pregnancy: Part I: Native Valves. *J. Am. Coll. Cardiol.* 46(2):223–230.

Thorne S.A. (2004) Pregnancy in heart disease. *Heart* 90(4):450–456.

Chapter 16 Infective endocarditis

Prendergast B. (2002) Diagnosis of infective endocarditis. *Brit. Med. J.* 32:845–846.

Prendergast B. (2006) The changing face of infective endocarditis. *Heart* 92:879–885.

Beynon R. (2006) Infective endocarditis. *Brit. Med. J.* 33:334–339.

Tornos P. (2005) Infective endocarditis in Europe - lessons from the Euro heart survey. *Heart* 91:571–575.

Index